BIOHARMONIC SELF-MASSAGE

BIOHARMONIC
SELF-MASSAGE

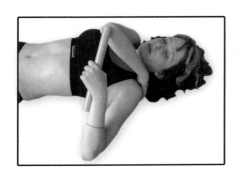

How to Harmonize
Your Mental, Emotional,
and Physical Energies

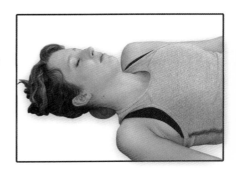

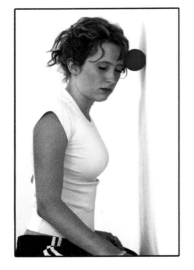

YVES BLIGNY

Translated by Jon E. Graham

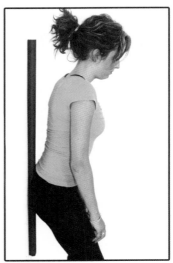

Healing Arts Press
Rochester, Vermont • Toronto, Canada

Healing Arts Press
One Park Street
Rochester, Vermont 05767
www.HealingArtsPress.com

Healing Arts Press is a division of Inner Traditions International

Originally published in French under the title *Automassages bioharmoniques: À la recontre de soi* by Éditions Jouvence
First U.S. edition published in 2011 by Healing Arts Press

Note to the reader: *This book is intended as an informational guide. The remedies, approaches, and techniques described herein are meant to supplement, and not to be a substitute for, professional medical care or treatment. They should not be used to treat a serious ailment without prior consultation with a qualified health care professional.*

Library of Congress Cataloging-in-Publication Data

Bligny, Yves.
  [Automassages bioharmoniques. English]
  Bioharmonic self-massage : how to harmonize your mental, emotional, and physical energies / Yves Bligny ; translated by Jon E. Graham. — 1st u.s. ed.
      p. cm.
  Includes bibliographical references and index.
  ISBN 978-1-59477-387-7 (pbk.)
  1. Massage therapy. I. Title.
  RM721.B6413 2011
  613.7'2—dc22

                                                                        2011009988

Printed and bound in India by Replika Press Pvt. Ltd.

10   9   8   7   6   5   4   3   2   1

Text design by Priscilla H. Baker; text layout by Virginia Scott Bowman
This book was typeset in Garamond Premier Pro with Gill Sans, Futura, and Arial Rounded as display typefaces
Model: Lora Bligny

CONTENTS

PART TWO
Practical Work

• • • • • • • •

I dedicate this book to my father,

to the grandfathers I never knew,

to the men of my family line,

most particularly those who were discreet,

too discreet!

ACKNOWLEDGMENTS

First and foremost I would like to gratefully thank Éditions Jouvence, and Jacques Maire in particular, for the confidence they have placed in me by providing this opportunity to share my ideas.

My personal and professional journey has crossed paths with many different people who have helped me expand and perfect my still evolving understanding.

My thoughts turn to the many individuals who have consulted me about their health problems. These encounters have always been a rich and challenging source of personal development.

My thoughts also turn prominently to the masseur and kinesiotherapist Georges Courchinoux. Our professional exchanges over the last fifteen years have improved and enhanced my work considerably, and I would like to acknowledge here my deep gratitude to him.

I would also like to thank all the teachers and researchers whose lectures and conferences I've attended, and whose books I have read, especially those who have most deeply marked and influenced me:

- Gerda Alexander, creator of Eutonie, who unstintingly gave me her support for the four years I was her neighbor. Her research, which should be better known, is still a great source of inspiration for me.
- Jean Emile Charon, Johann Soulas, Gerda Boyesen, and Marie Lise Labonté, all highly talented teachers and researchers.
- Dr. Ryke Geerd Hamer and all the other pioneers who upset popular wisdom and challenged hidebound beliefs, often at the price of their own lives or freedom.

- Sri Aurobindo and the Mother, both of whom were exceptional beings. The thirteen volumes of *The Mother's Agenda* are always a source of contemplation and inspiration for me.

I cannot overlook my wife, "a flawless mirror," who was constant in her support and assistance to me during the long period spent writing this book.

I would also like to give a quick nod to my brother Pat for his encouragement, and an even longer one to my mother.

My thanks to Mathias Plessis and to my daughter Lora for the photos, as well as to Françoise Morninière for her invaluable advice concerning the writing of this book.

Thanks to Claire just for being "herself."

In closing, I would like to thank that one thing without which nothing would exist and for which with every passing day my admiration and respect grow larger: life.

INTRODUCTION

A short excursion . . . for the purpose of finding yourself, through the path offered by your own body.

How I've Advanced on This Path

I have long regarded the body as a source of health and balance. Many extraordinary meetings have marked out the path of my personal and professional development, meetings that allowed me to experience the various dimensions of the body more deeply, to encounter other ways of living, and to increase my understanding of the fundamental oneness of being.

Through my practice and education, I have continued to deepen this insight and the research it has generated on the synergy between the body, emotions, thoughts, energy, consciousness, and brain.

My interests led to my initiation into a variety of therapeutic approaches, each of which shed new light and offered me a new "landscape," although there was none to which I could commit myself fully. One person says red, another says black, while yet another says white. As you can see, it is hard not to go astray in this terrain. Who can you trust? How can you find your way when you are not a professional?

Diversifying your approaches can cause you to scatter your energies unproductively as a kind of jack-of-all-trades, without any conductive thread. On the other hand, if you regard these approaches as different but complementary points of view and levels of one same reality, they can provide the optimum conditions for achieving the kind of open mind that inspires humility and great hope. These varied approaches make it possible to solidly plant your own practice in such a way that it can work synergistically with others.

Over time I realized that all the various trainings I'd received were like the pieces of a jigsaw puzzle that were falling into place, a puzzle whose end result remained a mystery to me but which was taking on a more definite form with the addition of each piece. Bioharmony was born of these various practices and my research—which is not to say that it is simply a synthesis of a lot of other approaches! It feeds on different domains of consciousness (particularly the neurosciences, quantum physics, and complex relativity), and it is inspired by the work of the Mother and Sri Aurobindo on the awakening of consciousness in matter.

The Approach

Bioharmony is an approach to holistic health and self-realization through the awakening of the body's consciousness and its natural potential to harmonize and free energy by releasing tensions and emotional memories. This bioharmonic approach offers us the opportunity to open our bodies to the life (in its sensorial, emotional, energetic, and memorial aspects) that is indwelling. A person on this path has no foes to battle and no adversaries to counter (no boundaries, resistances, or stiffness), just wonderful things to rediscover.

The emphasis here is on going deep within and learning to be receptive to sensations and feelings as catalysts for the body's bioharmonic potentials. This approach is supported by such practices as conscious-touch self-massage, different kinds of movements, nonverbal communication, corporeal expression, postures, stretches, and so forth.

This book offers an original and unprecedented way of performing self-massage with the help of balls, rollers, tubes, and different-sized rods or wands. As the result of many years of experimentation and practical application, these massages offer several advantages:

- They allow you to make contact *with all parts of your body.* In self-massage dependent upon the hands, many areas are impossible to reach or can be touched only through acrobatic contortions that are incompatible with the correct execution of the movements.
- These massages can be performed without strenuous effort and without causing fatigue, thanks to the simple use of the different tools in combination with the body's movements and its own weight.

- They make it easier for a person to remain in a state of openness and to simply let go.

These self-massages can be performed by anyone. They can easily be performed at home every day to soothe pain, release tension, decompress, get settled, empty the mind, relax the legs, balance energy, reduce stress levels, and stimulate awareness of the body and its sensations.

These techniques will be particularly valuable to healthcare professionals and to those leading physical education classes, gentle gymnastics classes, or relaxation groups. The work of all such people can be enriched with the addition of this simple and effective tool.

The practical part of this book offers many massage protocols for achieving more consistent balance of both mind and body, for staying healthy, and for relieving many problems of daily life. Every subject examined here is looked at from a theoretical, synthetic, and objective perspective. The exercises are explained in detail and accompanied by photos and illustrations so that they can be put into practice easily and correctly.

This book opens with a theoretical section. This is for the purpose of inviting readers to expand their understanding of the way they look at their corporeal reality and the synergy that exists between their body, energy, sensations, brain, and consciousness, as well as the potential for well-being that conscious awareness of their own body can bring them. Here I touch upon the following points: the psychosomatic dimension, the somatopsychic dimension, the profound oneness of every individual, the concept of energy, the bioharmonic process, holistic health, the importance of conscious intention, the different aspects of the body, and psycho-emotional recordings.

The Conductive Thread

My purpose in the first part of this book is to expand your knowledge about the psychosomatic (or somatopsychic) functioning of human beings and the profound unity or oneness of each individual being. This knowledge can help you to have a better understanding, or consciousness, of what you think, what you believe, and what you believe you have understood. You may not find everything you hope to find here, but one thing is sure: you will never find what you do not think or believe you can find.

Based on this expanded understanding and knowledge, we are able to provide our work with a meaning, a conductive thread. This allows us to perform our gestures with a clearer, wider intent, which in turn will allow us to work more deeply and more effectively.

This intention will necessarily rely upon various means and tools. In the context of self-massage, these tools are the simple objects (balls, tubes, wands, et cetera) that I call my true friends, my mirror objects.

And how do we do it? That is something we shall look at in the second part of the book. But first let's take a stroll on the paths to wisdom!

· · · · · · · ·

PART ONE

Theory

Knowledge and Understanding of Bioharmonics

1 • THE PSYCHOSOMATIC HUMAN

How the Mind Works upon the Body

Psyche: From the Greek *psukhe*, soul (*psukhikos,* the mind). That which is related to mind and consciousness; to a certain extent, that part of the being that engenders and governs our feelings and emotions.

Soma: From the Greek *soma,* the body. In biology this term refers to all the cells making up the body.

A Brief History of Psychosomatics

The term *psychosomatic* was first used by the German psychiatrist J. C. Henroth in his description of the origins of insomnia. The English psychiatrist Daniel Hack wrote the first manual of psychological medicine attesting to the mind's effect upon the body in 1872. His observations did not provide a systematic theoretical framework that could be used to mount a practical and effective treatment, and ignorance about the psychophysiological nature of emotions made it difficult to integrate Hack's observations into the new scientific medicine being developed in the nineteenth century. Rudolf Virchow's doctrine of cellular pathology, Louis Pasteur's and Robert Koch's doctrine of disease-causing germs, and the major discoveries then being made in the fundamental medical sciences (microbiology and biochemistry) combined to give the impression that disease was a product of faulty biomechanisms and primarily focused attention on the failings of the defective organ system.

Nevertheless, in the background, overshadowed by this dominant trend, events were transpiring that would eventually give birth to a new approach consisting of mind-body therapies. The phenomenon of conversion hysteria was made famous by Sigmund Freud (1856–1939), describing how a mental state transforms itself into a symbolic physical symptom, in this case a form of hysterical paralysis. Georg Groddeck (1836–1934) extrapolated the hypothesis of conversion with his suggestion that a disease's symptoms had an unconscious and symbolic meaning whose nature only the patient could unearth. Groddeck confirmed that once the patient became aware of this meaning, the symptoms inevitably disappeared, as they were no longer necessary.

For a twenty-year period beginning in 1940, Franz Alexander and his colleagues at the Chicago Institute for Psychoanalysis oversaw a vast study on the seven most common disorders whose physical causes were poorly understood. This research, followed by increasingly numerous studies on the psychophysiology of emotions, gave birth to the field of psychosomatic medicine.

According to Alexander, the primary cause of these seven disorders resided within an intrapsychic conflict whose origin could be located in earliest childhood. Such psychogenic influences are the frontiers of psychosomatic medicine.

Though most often ignored by twentieth-century medicine, today psychosomatic science is again recognized for what it is: "the study of the interactions of physical and psychosocial factors in the maintenance of health and the causation of disease." It so happens that the researchers of the last few years who have extensively studied the origins of physical pathological states have discovered that all degenerative, infectious, allergic, and autoimmune disorders can have their origin in the mind. This extremely hopeful development has taken the name of psychoneuroimmunology. One of these researchers, Professor Bernard Herzog, has published a book in which he makes a point of underscoring what is now for him and many others an incontestable scientific fact: the disorders of the soul induce physical diseases. What psychosomatics expresses, therefore, is that there is a reciprocal connection between the body (soma) and the psyche.

"It's psychosomatic!" When someone says this, he is saying everything and nothing. What's the next step? What do I mean when I speak of a connection? It is important to clearly and concretely grasp what forms this connection and to identify how and at what levels it expresses itself. It should be studied deeply enough so that it does not remain a simple piece of information (which I take into account only when it suits me) but is recognized as a realization that transforms something inside me, in my way of understanding things, and in my way of doing things and behaving.

I would like to try, using a number of simple examples based on recent research in the neurosciences and physics, to convince your rational Cartesian mind of this and to make you actually feel this connection and how complex it is at all its various levels.

We will start with the more obvious examples, obvious because they are based on experience and feeling, and go toward the less obvious, which are less evident only because they are unconscious or because their existence is not perceived as a possibility.

The Deliberate Decision

I count to three, and at the number three I raise one of my arms.

In this case my action is thought out; I've made up my mind to perform something and then acted upon it. My body is the performer of my will here. My movement in this case is the result of a conscious and considered decision.

Chronologically speaking, the mind intervenes before the soma.

Thought Inscribed within the Body

When you are buried in your thoughts, your body assumes a certain position: your face tends to freeze in place to a certain extent, and your eyes are either tightly focused in concentration or seem to be staring into space and drifting in the clouds.

On seeing you an outside observer will say, "She is deep in thought!" If this observer is quite attentive, he will see that your expression and posture subtly change in accordance with the flow of your thoughts (for example, the position of your eyes is constantly shifting).

The thought process is not a self-contained phenomenon that is amputated from your body; you are not able to think without a body. The mechanism of thought exists concretely only because it is inscribed within a cerebro-muscular process.

Note: Being constantly lost in thought, or "too much in your head," as they say, is evidence of an imbalance on the physiological, muscular, circulatory level. From an energetic perspective, it "overloads" the top and empties the bottom.

Emotion Inscribed in the Body

This connection between the emotions and the body is felt clearly only under certain circumstances. When I am in the grip of an emotion, generally speaking, I can feel it inside and I can name it. If my awareness of the moment is broader (as would be the case for thought), I might be able to feel its external inscription in my muscle tone, through an attitude or an expression that could indicate to some outside observer that I am feeling sad, angry, beaten down, or whatever. But this inscription that is visible to others is one I do not often feel in my body.

If we were to analyze these different parameters, we would see changes (specific to the emotion) at the level of blood circulation, energy flow, and the function of the organs, and in sensations: heat, tingling, and so on.

Let's now observe an individual at these different levels. This state of being* manifests itself through:

- The feeling of the emotion (the self-contained emotion)
- Its muscular inscription (attitude, posture, facial expression)
- The state of the circulatory system, only at this moment, as well as the way the organs are functioning and so forth (autonomic nervous system and so on)
- Sensations (tensions, pains, lightheadedness, and so on)

A specific emotional state displays a unique coloration at these different levels, and *from the moment the emotion is no longer the same, the corporeal parameters are no longer the same.* It is a case of which comes first, the chicken or the egg? We will answer this question later.

Note: Here I am speaking about situations in which the psycho-emotional state is expressing and revising itself at center stage. But there are plenty of times when psycho-emotional states cannot fully express themselves and work themselves out. These are cases in which they have been interrupted at the beginning of their manifestation or even nipped in the bud. There can be multiple reasons for this interruption—social, educative, psychological, emotional, and so forth in nature.

---

*The state of being encompasses the individual's different levels of existence: physical, emotional, psychological, energetic, and so on.

These expressions are then shoved into the background: you can no longer feel them, see them, hear them; you are no longer aware of them and they are severed from you. But they are still there (as they have not completed expressing themselves). They have become inscribed within a cerebro-autonomic-muscular pattern and leave traces on different levels (biological, physiological, mechanical, muscular, energetic, and so on), thereby creating an imbalance.

In the first example, where there is a conscious and deliberate decision, the psyche seems to be the *first* step in how the operation unfolds. The physical reactions are a consequence of the thought, like the pins struck by a bowling ball. "When I think of my angry boss, I feel scared and my stomach contracts."

In the other examples (thought, emotions), this chronology is not so obvious. There are popular expressions that perfectly express this connection between the mind and the body, between the inner state and what it manifests, such as "It took over my head!" or "It caught in my throat!"

Let's take another example to illustrate this relationship. This time we will consider a book.

First Level of Contact

It is an object that occupies a volume in space. I am able to describe it: it is made with paper pages and a cardboard cover. If I open it, I will see letters printed on its pages. My body, if I observe it externally, with my eyes or hands, similarly occupies a volume in space: it is limited by its skin and what it has beneath this skin—muscles, bones, and organs, which I can more or less feel.

Second Level of Contact

If I hold this book, I will feel its texture, its thickness, the elasticity of its cover, its pages, its aroma, and so on. This body, if I take the time to tune into it and open up to it, will display the appearance of sensations: the heat in my hands, my cold feet, a small sensation of tension in my back, and so on.

Third Level of Contact

Let's now turn the pages of our book and enter the story that has been recorded in it. We find ourselves embarking into an *inner space,* made up of sentiments, actions, emotions, landscapes, and suspense. This story, whose plot unfurls inside places that I can imagine and even feel, is one that I capture and contact through a space defined three-dimensionally (the inner space), made of cardboard, paper, and letters that carry a meaning. If I can make myself receptive to the latter, I can then grasp the story.

It is the same thing for a computer disk (equivalent to the body, or soma). I can break it into tiny pieces and still never find its inner space, and yet once I insert this disk inside a computer, this inner space (equivalent to the mind, or psyche) will manifest and become tangible through the screen.

To Recap

Your emotion (joy, fear, sorrow, or some other) is not just an inner state, a self-contained emotion. It is both the container (the corporeal dimension) and the content (inner space). It exists and lives because it is inscribed in your flesh. Touch the buttocks of someone in the street with your hand and you shall definitely see that the gluteal muscle (which is made up of tendons and fibers) is not just an anatomical element! For now it is important to grasp that the soma (body) and the psyche (mind) are two dimensions that cannot be separated and are always together.

In this first psychosomatic component, I have tried to show by means of concrete examples that when the psyche (the emotional state, the affective mind) changes, the soma also changes, and there are no thoughts or emotions that are not accompanied by physical phenomena.

---

2 • THE SOMATOPSYCHIC HUMAN

How the Body Works upon the Mind

The body in the broad sense of the word influences the psycho-emotional state. To be more specific, a change on the level of the body, which is chronologically first, is accompanied by a change in the mind. In this case, it is the action upon the body by means of the body that comes first. Next, and sometimes almost instantaneously, thought and emotion appear.

As in the first chapter, we shall start by looking at the most obvious cases, where the functioning involved is easy to grasp, and then proceed to examine the more subtle connections.

Everyone has had the experience of drinking a small glass of wine or beer and feeling good, a little less inhibited and more euphoric, feeling more free to act, as well as the experience of feeling the sorrow that alcohol sometimes induces.

Drugs have very powerful effects on the psycho-emotional plane. Laboratory experiments have shown that injecting certain chemical substances creates emotional states (fear, for example), without any external causes to trigger them.

These examples are obvious, but the ones that follow should raise questions about the mechanics of this connection between psyche and soma, between mind and body: egg or chicken?

Several Small Experiments

Stand up, then allow your head to fall forward, curve your back, slump your shoulders, and walk around the room. What do you feel taking place inside your body (tugging sensations, pain, pressure)? How do you feel personally? Joyous, happy, full of pep? What is the overall atmosphere?

Stand up straight again, and thrust your head forward, followed by your lower jaw, while tightly clenching your fists; now how do you feel? Is it the same way the previous exercise made you feel? What is your state of being? (You can play with this exercise indefinitely.)

Observe the way people walk. Some people have a very characteristic walk that gives you the impression that one part of the body is dragging the rest, but as a rule the dynamic is much more subtle and unique for each individual. Which part of the body is leading the way most prominently? Which part lags behind? Is it the head, shoulders, chest, belly, pelvis, or lower limbs?

Next watch one person, and try to imitate his or her way of walking, putting yourself in that person's skin and capturing his or her physical state and state of being.

A number of studies conducted by Professor Paul Ekman and his collaborators are very instructive. Their purpose was to establish this reciprocal and unbreakable connection between the cognitive brain and the emotional brain. To evaluate this connection, they asked their test subjects to contract their facial muscles in a certain sequence in such a way that unbeknownst to them their expression became one of joy, sorrow, or fear. They did not know what expression their face was displaying. They had no thought in their mind to cause the displayed emotion. Yet they all eventually felt the emotion that was represented by their expression.

The first examples (drink, drugs) show that by changing the body's chemistry through the intake of substances, the psycho-emotional state will change. What happens in this regard with food? How does the chemistry of our diet influence us psycho-emotionally? How much does it affect us? It is often said that you are what you eat. The Chinese offer a variation on this in their adage that you become what you eat!

The last example shows that when a change occurs in certain parameters of the body by virtue of an intentional, conscious action, a variation also occurs in the psycho-emotional state. Though the changes in the first cases were clear-cut and easily felt, there are others that can be more subtle and gradual, which cannot be felt and pass beneath the radar of our awareness (all the more so when we ignore them as a possibility).

These different experiments and recent research in neuroscience have given new fuel to somatopsychic approaches, by virtue of demonstrating that by acting out of and upon the body, we can also affect the psyche.

In his book *Looking for Spinoza: Joy, Sorrow, and the Feeling Brain*, Antonio R. Damasio, a great neurologist with a worldwide reputation, revisits the bond and mechanisms shared by emotions and feelings. In an interview with neuroscientist, author, and physician David Servan-Schreiber in *Psychologies* magazine, Damasio said:

> What we experience mentally is always the result of corporeal changes, by changing our body's state, we change our way of perceiving everything that happens to us, our perception of the world. By helping the body become physiologically healthier, we can influence the way we experience our feelings and emotions. By learning more about our emotions, in physiological terms, we are able to develop a daily effect on our body's experience in such a way that lets us lead a happier life.

These are truly important discoveries that are able to enlighten us and expand the practice of psychotherapy and medicine in general! In that same interview Damasio went on to say:

> When you feel a deep pain or great sorrow over a prolonged period of time, the implications go beyond the mind to affect what we call the body. This is the same body that is treated by medicine or surgery.
>
> These emotional states can have consequences on the immune system and breed infections or contribute to the development of cancer.
>
> This is something that is fairly well known and yet it has had almost no impact in medicine. We continue to treat cancer, infections, and heart disease as if these conditions were exclusively physical, without evaluating, first, the mental impact of the disease, and, second, what the mind has done to create this disease and will continue doing unless this action is identified and resolved.
>
> I think that the medical system needs to be turned upside down, whether it is pulmonology, infectious diseases, cardiology, rheumatology, or dermatology. None of these domains can be grasped and fully understood without taking

into account the patient's frame of mind, the regulating element of his brain, and his or her autonomic nervous system.

Everything is influenced by these systems . . . I do not think we can move forward if we continue separating the body from the mind, as is [the] current standard operating procedure . . .

To begin understanding these relations in neuro-scientific terms, I suggest the idea of a "body map," in other words the depiction of our body in our brain. We could picture it a little like a dashboard that is constantly being updated with information on the state of every organ and physiological function.

To Recap

We have seen that depending on certain situations and certain moments, it is sometimes the egg (the psyche) and sometimes the chicken (the soma) that comes first.

Whether it is in the psychosomatic or the somatopsychic sense, the body, emotions, feelings, and thoughts are permanently interrelated.

There is no mental activity (thoughts, feelings, emotions) that is unaccompanied by constant changes in the body (muscle tone, blood circulation, hormonal secretions).

There are no changes in the body that are not echoed in the mind (feelings, thoughts, emotions). The brief experiments I've suggested for you to try will make this easier to grasp. For the hardened Cartesian rationalist, the most recent research in neuroscience can confirm this beyond question.

How does this (neurological, hormonal, energetic) connection work? Am I trembling because I am scared? Or am I scared because I am trembling?

3 • WHAT COMES FIRST, THE CHICKEN OR THE EGG?

But just what is this body-mind connection? How do we experience and understand it?

Is this bond at work when an emotion brings about a certain muscular contraction? Is this contraction the consequence of the emotion, like the bowling pin that falls at the impact of the ball that just struck it?

How can we grasp this concept, and how can we experience this event at a given moment? Should we perceive the psyche and the soma as separate pieces that interact with each other, like a ball that knocks down a pin that in turn knocks down others as it falls? Is this interaction a chronology of events that can be expressed algebraically, for example, using the letter T to express the variable of time represented by a given moment: T, T + 1, T + 2?

Are you trembling because you are scared, or are you scared because you are trembling? If you stopped trembling, would your fear go away?

Couldn't we shift into a new paradigm of understanding? This new paradigm would involve the realization that we function synergistically, that there is no cause-and-effect interaction at work between the mind and body, and that the body, emotions, and feelings are only *aspects of one same reality,* that they form an entity whose parts are unified by their simultaneous and synergic mode of functioning.

We human beings are a functional and synergic whole. "This makes me feel bad" transforms into "I feel bad," thereby incorporating in one fell swoop the physical, emotional, and mental dimensions of the same experience.

It is extremely important to grasp this profound synergy: by touching your body with a certain intention and awareness, you are also making contact with your emotions and thoughts, and by encouraging their expression, you are also encouraging a physical transformation.

The Contribution of the Neurosciences

First, what are they telling us?

The Role of Emotions

For a long time emotions were not deemed worthy of being cited in research programs. Throughout the twentieth century, the neurosciences and cognitive sciences had become fixed to the study of the so-called superior processes of the human brain, such as the power to reason, language, calculation, and memory, comparing the brain's functioning to that of a computer. Obviously, a fixed notion of mental functioning like this created an impasse for considerations such as emotions, feelings, and the body. Moods, as Antonio R. Damasio put it, were a vague and unquantifiable notion.

But over the last twelve years, advances in neuroscience have scrapped the computer metaphor, replacing it with a much more dynamic vision of the brain, one that attributes an essential role to emotion.

New visualization techniques such as PET (positron-emission tomography—a branch of nuclear medicine imaging or NMI) and MRI (magnetic resonance imaging) now offer extremely powerful investigative tools. The brain concealed within its skull is gradually surrendering its secrets.

The Three Brains

- The most primitive, the reptilian brain (basically the brain stem and the cerebellum), is the center for primary instincts.
- The intermediary brain is that of the emotions (the limbic system).
- The most recent, the higher brain, also known as the neocortex, includes the envelope of the two hemispheres. It is the seat of language and thought.

The tissue of the limbic (emotional) brain is cruder and its neurons are amalgamated and not stacked in regular layers as they are in the neocortex. This configuration is more propitious for the rapid reactions that are necessary for survival.

The limbic brain is a command post that is constantly receiving information from the different parts of the body and responding to them appropriately by monitoring physiological equilibrium: respiration, cardiac rhythm, blood pressure, appetite, sleep, libido, the release of hormones, and immune system function.

From this viewpoint, our emotions are only the *conscious experience of a vast ensemble of physiological reactions, which are constantly supervising and making adjustments to the activity of the biological systems of the body as they confront the imperatives of the inner and outer environment.* The limbic brain is therefore almost on a more intimate footing with the body than with the neocortex. This is why it is often easier to gain access to emotions through the body than through speech.

As underscored by David Servan-Schreiber:

Our emotional brain is much more than a cumbersome vestige of our animal past: master of our bodies and our passions, it is the very source of our identity and the values that give meaning to our lives.

Descartes' Error

What have we learned from all the many investigations and observations of brains that have been damaged through accident or as a result of illness or degeneration?

The world-famous neuroscientist Antonio R. Damasio shows that the ability to reason is actually founded upon the emotions. One of his patients, a man named Elliot, was recovering quite well physically from the removal of a brain tumor. His high IQ had not been adversely affected, but he seemed to have lost the ability to make sensible decisions. He had the knowledge but not the know-how, Damasio explains. What was he now missing? Social emotions like sympathy, guilt, and shame, all of which he had ceased feeling since the time of his illness. Disconnected from emotional experience, his rational brain, although still completely intact, was now simply spinning its wheels.

What Damasio took from these fleeting signs—conscious and unconscious—that leave an imprint of our emotions in our bodies in such manifestations as blushing, butterflies in the stomach, and the feeling of one's heart in one's throat was the notion of the somatic marker. These intimate signals are "inserted" into the emotional brain and involuntarily surge up every time an analogous situation takes place, or even at the smallest occurrence that brings back to mind the circumstances that initially inspired these reactions.

Freud therefore had been correct in postulating the existence of repression and the unconscious, even if this does leave us a long way from Lacan's cherished "unconscious structured like a language."

So was Descartes wrong? Not only are the body and mind not independent, but his *Cogito ergo sum* (I think, therefore I am) points us in a wrong direction. *I feel my body, therefore I am,* would seem to be more appropriate.

Here is what Damasio has to say on this topic:

What we could consider as the most spiritual and most elevated aspects in our life could easily correspond with those physical states that define the ideal mechanism of the living being. You could call it the magic that hides behind life . . .

In the same way that anger or shame correspond to a particular configuration of the body, we can define a configuration of the body that could be labeled spiritual.

These states manifest in specific circumstances and attract specific thoughts. They are inspired by certain stimuli that arise from works of art by passing through nature . . . And the state that results is an incredible state of physiological harmony.

I compare the notion of the spiritual to an intense expression of harmony, to the feeling that the body has attained its most perfect level of functioning. This experience is accompanied by the desire to act toward others with compassion and generosity.

When I connect spiritual experiences to the neurobiology of feelings, I am not trying to reduce the sublime to mechanical and therefore cheapen its worth. I am rather trying to suggest that there is something sublime in the spiritual that is embodied in what is biologically sublime, and we can begin to grasp the underlying process in biological terms.

The fact of providing an explanation of the physiological processes at work behind the spiritual does not explain the mystery inherent in the life process to which this particular sentiment is attached. It reveals the bond it has with the mystery but not the mystery itself.

Spinoza Was Right

While Cartesian dualism makes an uneasy bedfellow with the neurosciences, Spinoza's monism, in which body and mind are two aspects of the same substance, is, in contrast, on the same wavelength.

In his book, Damasio hails Spinoza's brilliant intuitions, such as his famous concept of *conatus* (a kind of vital energy that the philosopher defines as the ceaseless effort made by all living organisms to ensure their self-preservation). He finds its physical expression in what he calls the congenital neurobiological wisdom of our brain, designed by evolution to help us manage the body.

The conatus, the natural effort of self-preservation, is automatically activated when confronted by suffering and death. Simply mentioning this perspective is enough to throw our physiological balance off-kilter; the conatus responds to this imbalance through emotional reactions that are almost reflexes, and beneficial, and which cause individuals to take action to ensure their survival, such as fleeing when danger threatens or dulling the sensation of pain when self-defense proves necessary.

Science confirms this: the best physician for all our ills is the body itself, thanks to its intrinsic ability to defend itself and restore homeostasis. Our emotions and feelings act as sentinels that alert our conscious ego to the state of our organism at any given moment.

Damasio shows that joyful states, whether truly felt or imaginary, correspond to these states of balance in the organism: physiological coordination is optimal, conditions for survival are at their most favorable, and well-being is foremost. In contrast, states of sorrow provoke a functional imbalance:

> We should seek joy, by reasoned decree, regardless of how foolish and unrealistic the quest may look. For the same reasons we should sever our connections with negative emotions like fear, anger, jealousy, and sorrow.

The Practical Consequences

Recent findings and research have shed additional light on and reinforced what the humanist psychologists of the 1960s were striving to accomplish with their therapies: reintegrating the body into the healing process and psychological health—this same body that Freud had excluded from the domain of curing in order to center the language of the quest [for healing] on the unconscious.

Several of Freud's disciples criticized him for this eviction and established dissident schools in which work on and through the body was used as a tool for harmonization and holistic health. Carl Gustav Jung, Wilhelm Reich, and Otto Rank were responsible for laying the groundwork for the rise of dozens of variations and methods grouped together under the label of psychocorporeal therapies, including primal scream, rebirthing, Gestalt, bioenergetics, postural integration, and so forth. Born in the effervescent atmosphere of the Californian counterculture, these imaginative, audacious, innovative, and sometimes exuberant therapies all have their benefits and flaws.

Over the course of time, these therapies have evolved (with better theoretical understanding and practice) and nurtured new ones, some of which stem directly from scientific discoveries validated by studies offering assurances of strictness and credibility, such as EMDR (eye movement desensitization and reprocessing) therapy and heart coherence.

Let's read what Damasio has to say in this regard:

We can think as much as we like that the mind arises from the brain, in other words . . . the body/mind split . . . on the one side we have the head made up of a brain-mind, and on the other, the body itself, . . . [but this] prevents understanding of the decisive role played by the body in things concerning the mind.

Soma and psyche are two faces of the same entity, but with a slight asymmetry that benefits the first: earlier to evolve, the body in fact models the contents of the mind more than the mind does its own contents.

Here is the position taken by Jack Painter, the creator of postural integration:

If any aspect of my experience is changed, all the others are as well. I am not saying that one part of me influences this or that other part, for example, [a relaxing] of muscular tension affects my thoughts and emotions: the relaxation of physical tension is [a] relaxing of emotional or mental frustrations, just as the release of these frustrations is [the release] of my physical tensions. We can look at the body as a functional aspect of emotions and thought, and these latter can be seen as a function of the body; by working on the body, you are already working on the mind, and vice versa . . . The practitioner knows that by touching the body, superficially or deeply, he is also making contact with emotions and thoughts and by encouraging [their expression], he is also encouraging a physical transformation.

From a therapeutic perspective, two decisive consequences emerge from this observation:

- Among the most effective methods are those that rely upon the organism's ability to heal itself through the implementation of a self-regulating force, a force that is far beyond the grasp of our knowledge and intelligence.
- The resolution of disorders is achieved through the harmony of the emotional brain, the cognitive brain, and the physiology of the body.

Says Damasio:

It's a new world of healing opening up before the field of medicine. In several years, we will realize how much more effective preventive measures are than chemistry. We will treat pain, psychosomatic disorders, mental problems with made-to-order treatments based on nutrition, exercise, psychocorporeal exercises, with medication playing a complementary role that is adapted on a case-by-case basis.

Psychiatrists like David Servan-Schreiber are already working on this neo-holistic approach that has been shaped by scientific advances. Their courage and clairvoyance should be saluted in the current ultrafragmented state of medicine, where every specialist clings tightly to a specialty.

A movement is already well under way in the United States. It is now known as mind-body medicine. Its leader is Professor Jim Gordon, former chairman of the White House Commission on Complementary and Alternative Medicine Policy. He often travels to war-torn nations to train professional healers there in many tried and tested methods borrowed from traditional medicines such as self-hypnosis, meditation, acupuncture, osteopathy, herbal medicine, and so forth. His staff at the Center for Mind-Body Medicine offers group therapies for individuals suffering from chronic conditions such as cancer, cardiovascular disease, depression, anxiety, and so forth.

Could the reconciliation of science with the empiricism of the oldest healing traditions be currently under way? This would be incredibly good news if true.

To Recap

Neuroscience provides us with illumination on the mechanism of this connection between mind and body, through the support provided by the nervous system and the hormonal system, on the profound oneness of its functioning. It also shows us that, in any event, manifested life cannot be experienced (thoughts, emotions, feelings, sensations) without a nervous system, without the body.

Like a tree, the apple can only exist thanks to roots, soil, a trunk, branches, and flowers. The fruit could never come into existence without all that, and its quality depends in large part upon these different elements.

A caterpillar is not a butterfly, but without a caterpillar there will be no butterfly.

Whether it is the egg or the chicken that comes first, the other is ever present. One cannot exist without the other. The question to ask may not be "Which comes first, the chicken or the egg?" but "What is the origin of the process that lies behind the chicken and the egg?"

It is quite simply life itself, the source of everything, from the most basic cell to the most sophisticated creation yet achieved by nature: the human being.

This life by definition is constantly manifesting, continuing to live, maintaining itself, and flowering, particularly through harmonizing regulatory processes. Scientists such as Antonio Damasio speak of this manifestation in terms of congenital neurobiological wisdom, psychocorporeal therapies, life intelligence, biodynamic life force, and so on, and the philosophy of conatus, the unique substance located at the origin of our thoughts, our emotions, and all the reactions of our body.

Experiments and research have also shown us that the body and the mind are one unit, two faces of a single piece. Our thoughts, our emotions, and our physical functions are the diverse facets of the different levels of manifestation of one single phenomenon: life.

We cannot avoid making an analogy with the Eastern traditions, in which the body and psyche are seen as different levels of energy, the source of life and its manifestations. The disturbance and disrupted balance of this energy is expressed by a group of mental and physical symptoms (even the strongest manifestation of this imbalance is sometimes physical, sometimes mental), which are the "colorations" of these different levels on which the disrupted energy is manifested.

Everyone is expressing, in accordance with their approach and by using different words, the same thing. This is that same thing that animates all of us and has created us to be so intelligent: life! (And as it exceeds our ability to understand it by means of our intelligence, it is a good idea to put our trust in it.) It is life, or energy.

We find ourselves entering a domain that is incredibly complicated but also exceedingly rich. It is one that can enrich the perspective of the neurosciences, help us put our convictions into perspective, expand our horizons and our understanding of the mind and body, and give us more hope and possibilities in our unending quest for well-being.

Follow me if you wish to learn more of this domain. We are about to make a quick tour of the fundamental branch of science known as physics.

The Perspective of Physics

Energy

The word *energy* comes from the Greek words *en* and *ergon,* which literally mean "in action."

"I am full of energy," "I don't have the energy left to do this or that," "the energy of despair"—in all these common expressions, this word *energy* refers to this something, a source, an origin, a motor for action, for starting things off, for realization. But the term encompasses a vast number of notions, domains, and levels.

I have the modest ambition of casting some light on the landscape of this energy through what I've been able to learn, grasp, and experience. Present at every moment in our daily life, it proves to be one of those things that everyone talks about constantly but rarely ever sees, except for those times when it is made luminous.

Everything is energy! Science itself confirms it.

From the smallest living organism to the largest, from a single grain of sand to a solar system, everything is definitively composed of elementary particles known as atoms. An atom consists of a nucleus and electron(s) that gravitate around that nucleus, much as planets gravitate around the sun in a solar system. It is not easy to depict an atom or its size. If I were to enlarge one atom one thousand billion times, the nucleus would become a dot one centimeter in diameter, the electron or electrons would be around 1 to 2 millimeters in diameter, and the distance separating them would be around 1 kilometer, or a little more than half a mile. Each atom is therefore about 99.999 percent emptiness and contains only the merest trace of matter.

If we were to remove the empty space between the nuclei and the electrons, all the atoms that make up our Earth could be held in a thimble, but one whose weight would be equivalent to that of the entire planet!

By the same token, this book you are reading, the chair in which you are sitting, and the solid ground holding you up are formed by almost nothing but emptiness, and yet this emptiness is quite solid. This solidity comes from the fact that between the nuclei and the electrons, there are forces directly connected with different energies. These energies connect the nuclei together in such a way that your chair does not collapse and your body does not break down into a thousand pieces.

Energy and an unimaginably small trace of matter (the nucleus and the electron): this was basically all that I had retained, like most others who took physics in school. So let's keep moving forward . . .

The numerous particles at the origin of the universe—of life and its various aspects (animal, vegetable, mineral, human)—all interact (are in relationship with one another) in a diverse manner (infinitely large or infinitely small), and they are all to some extent descriptions of the different properties of energy.

We make a distinction between:

- Electromagnetic interactions
- Weak interactions, which are responsible for some decays of nuclear particles
- Strong interactions, which ensure the coherence of the protons and neutrons that bind together to form the nuclei of atoms
- Gravitational interactions, primarily the force of gravity that "glues" us to the ground

Science has sought to find the unifying factor for all these various physical phenomena. This unification project is accompanied by theoretical and experimental research on the structure of the most elementary forms of matter. Analysis of matter particles placed inside increasingly powerful accelerators has made it possible to discover even more elementary particles.

Physicists have therefore found agreement on the notion that as long as one is dealing with material particles occupying a spatial volume that is not a void, such particles cannot be considered to be anything but punctual particles, in other words particles that are represented in the physical space of our universe as veritable mathematical points, each point being, by definition, a zero spatial volume.

It was this strictly punctual aspect of the most elementary particles appearing in the formation of matter that became increasingly evident in physics research conducted during the 1960s and 1970s. Thus, starting in the 1970s, physics had established the presence of matter particles characterized by a punctual volume, a subjective psi wave (characteristic of extrasensory perception and other paranormal phenomena) that spread in an infinite distance and at an infinite rate of speed around the particle under examination, and by a set of numbers representing the purely abstract properties of the point particle.

By the end of the 1970s, physics had managed to empty the entire space of our universe of its material content, at least in a certain way. All that remained were points of no volume, subjective psi waves, and whole numbers associated to abstract properties. Could this be what Eastern thought had in mind when it told us the world was naught but an illusion?

In the decade of the 1980s, work still remained necessary to fully realize the great unification. This was a period during which science opened up the space of the universe to hidden dimensions: the 1983 Nobel Prize–winning work of physicist Abdus Salam on supergravity, the superstring theory that won John Schwarzen the Nobel Prize in 1985 . . . But the unification had not been achieved in any thorough or coherent fashion. Both Salam's and Schwarzen's models dealt only with the question of space, unlike what Einstein had realized. *It was necessary to introduce a new aspect of time.*

A certain number of scientists did make this leap and began speaking of another hidden dimension in which *the benchmarks for time, space, and speed are different.* Each (mathematical) point that represents each particle of matter is only a kind of punctual trace of something that stretches out in space. But it is a different space, a place that is "somewhere else" but still remains a part of our entire universe (for more, see appendix 1).

Consciousness and Energy

Inside his framework of complex relativity, Jean E. Charon posits the existence in the universe of a total space-time that includes:

- Ordinary reality, consisting of a cosmological time and a cosmological space
- The imaginal realm, a space-time continuum that is made up (in every point of reality) of four additional dimensions, whose base vectors are those of reality

The following diagram furnishes the representation of a particle of matter as proposed by complex relativity.

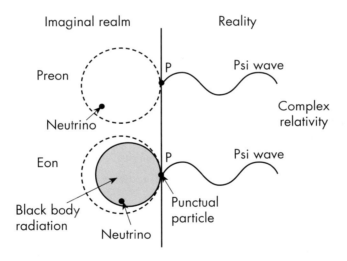

A particle of matter therefore simultaneously extends over both reality and the imaginal realm, in which the symbols of its memory (sigma field) reside.

This fundamental criterion distinguishes an artificial memory, like that in a computer, from the individual memory. There is nothing hidden in the computer memory; everything is in the space it occupies. All its points, both hardware and software,* are in real space. It is true that the computer program needs to be interpreted in order to be understood, not by the computer itself but by a third

---

*Computer memories

party, generally a human being, who has knowledge about the program. A computer by itself would be unusable and useless. It would serve no purpose.

There is another primary difference between individual living memory and that of a computer. The former, unlike the latter, not only knows, but knows that it knows, hence the notion of mind or consciousness.

During the years 1955–1960, the neurophysiologist John Eccles (who won the Nobel Prize for medicine in 1963) put forth the idea that the brain was only a simple computer that transmitted information. The system software and the programming were located somewhere else. He ventured the hypothesis that a particle field existed that had not yet been detected by the instruments of physicists. This field was the exact program and system software of the brain. By coordinating them, the cortex transmits the information it receives from the material field of the mind. What it is, in fact, is the primary model of material consciousness.

This was followed by numerous models of consciousness such as the fundamental ideas of Karl Pribam and David Bohm, which involved a veritable paradigm shift (benchmarks, references), an entirely new notion of the universe associated with a model of consciousness. These two scientists followed two different courses of research yet reached the same conclusion.

Initially a neurosurgeon, Karl Pribam thought that what we called reality was only a holographic projection of a *fundamental universe,* which he called the frequency domain, in which time and space have both collapsed and all that exists are waves, which Pribam places in a different dimension.

In this frequency domain, all events exist without any connotation of time and space. The interface of consciousness and the cortex are capable of analyzing all the interference patterns from this domain and projecting them in the form of holograms into a system of arbitrary coordinates that we call time and space. From this standpoint, the stars, the galaxy, particles, and living creatures are only holograms, as is the entire visible universe.

While they are formulated in a different language—speaking in terms of the implicate and explicate orders—the ideas of David Bohm are entirely comparable to those of Pribam.

Régis Dutheil speaks of a *subluminous* and a *superluminous* world. His reasoning is based on a model of superluminous consciousness, in which consciousness is a field of tachyonic matter. This field forms part of the true fundamental universe of which our world is only a subluminous holographic projection.

Dutheil constructed a model of superluminous material consciousness formed by a superluminous matter that is made up of particles known as tachyons, which travel faster than the speed of light. These tachyons are connected to a different space-time continuum than the subluminous one that governs our world.

In superluminous space-time, time and space no longer have the same qualities. Time itself, as we experience it, becomes spatial and no longer flows (!!??), which corresponds to the concept of an infinite speed. To a tachyonic observer there is no longer any past, present, or future, and all events exist in a way that is both instantaneous and yet enduring.

Furthermore, whereas in our subluminous universe flowing time corresponds to the growth of entropy, which means that we travel from a situation of order to one of increasing disorder (the only means of fighting against this growth is with information), in the superluminous universe, to the contrary, entropy is constantly shrinking: information and meaning are in a permanent state of increase.

For Dutheil, consciousness or the mind consists of a field of tachyons or superluminous matter, located *on the other side of the wall of light* in superluminous space-time. Taking up Bohm's and Pribam's ideas again, Dutheil used Pribam's frequency domain to form his superluminous universe, which is also reminiscent of Jean E. Charon's imaginal realm.

According to Dutheil, our subluminous universe is nothing but the holographic projection of the fundamental universe consisting of information and meaning. This projection is carried out by means of an electrical field, which acts as a filter and only allows a very small portion of information and meaning to pass into the flow of entropic time. We could say that there is an intermediary physical system ensuring the projection of the holograms that we ourselves are. In great likelihood this system is an electromagnetic field whose existence seems to have been solidly established by Harold Saxton Burr.

Burr's Vital Field

Harold S. Burr, a professor of anatomy at Yale University, enthusiastically pursued a course of research over a forty-year span, with the help of a team of biologists and physicists. He provided indisputable evidence of an electromagnetic field that surrounds all living organisms, including human beings. I will not go into great detail about his experiments but simply summarize the important points and characteristics of this field.

One essential characteristic of this field is that it varies over the course of time in response to a group of internal and external factors (according to quantum physics, the particles associated with an electromagnetic field are photons that move at the speed of light). What are they?

An enormous increase in voltage was observed during a twenty-four-hour period occurring around once a month. This change corresponded to the midway point of the menstrual cycle (with laboratory-confirmed ovulation in studies using female rabbits).

These field variations were studied by Burr and his successors, particularly Leonard Ravitz, who demonstrated (in gynecology) that this field showed a disturbance before symptoms of a disease became clinical or even manifested themselves anatomopathologically. This allows us to believe that the same would hold true for every pathological syndrome. What a valuable tool for making an early diagnosis!

Measured over long periods of time, this field revealed the presence of regular cycles indicative of the times when the individual felt at tip-top form and those times when his or her vitality was diminished.

The Burr field comes into existence with ovulation and can even be recorded in unfertilized eggs. It is therefore a primordial field in which the interactions observed between the physical organs and this electromagnetic field within the organism are only subsequent occurrences.

Like iron filings that arrange themselves in accordance with the lines of force specific to the magnetic field of the magnet, Burr has shown evidence through his study of salamanders that the cells of the embryo are assembled in accordance *with the pattern of an electromagnetic field that preexists the birth of the salamander.*

The field's influence on chromosome data, in other words on genetic programming, has been proven with other experiments. One in particular seems to demonstrate that chromosomes and therefore DNA molecules can use this field to transmit a blueprint or a change in the blueprint to the protoplasm. Burr successfully read the electromagnetic blueprint to establish a distinction between two kinds of corn before their differences had become visible.

Edward Russell envisions this vital field as an integrative mechanism that not only provides the model for the organism but survives its biological death. Whatever the case may prove to be, the vital field is a kind of exact electronic image of the body, in which certain details can appear before they can be detected physically.

A living structure therefore consists of two systems: the soma and the vital (or electromagnetic) field.

The work of Robert O. Becker, specialist in orthopedic surgery, also provides confirmation of the existence of this vital field. He gave particular study to the problem of the joining of fractured limbs (which is especially difficult among the elderly). Many of Becker's experiments were performed on frogs and salamanders. Among these latter, the electrical potentials diminished rapidly at the time the limb was amputated, then suddenly began rising again until they reached a level three times higher than their initial level. After several weeks, the regeneration process began and a new limb began forming.

Using this observation as his starting point, Becker experimented with several different kinds of electrical current at fracture sites, which produced some spectacular results in the treatment of serious injuries. In these same conditions, he was able to stave off infection, provide pain relief, restore muscular control and the intestinal wall, and regenerate nerves. His work clearly shows the existence of an electromagnetic body, which we are just beginning to take into consideration.

From the mechanical perspective, Becker has shown that when an organism produces electrical currents or fields, it forms semiconductive systems possessing very interesting properties. This system transmits only a weak current, but it does so at a high speed when the temperature rises, and it can transmit the current great distances.

Inorganic crystals such as silicon have semiconductivity as a natural property. Every time a current traverses silicon, the crystal alters its structure, which enables the current to pass through more easily the next time, and so on (the property of hysteresis). Silicon crystals bear a strong resemblance to living substances. Like all tissues, nerve tissue includes proteins. If they behave like semiconductors, they, too, would be extremely sensitive to the signals sent by this electric field.

The Kirlian Effect

Kirlian photographs are images of a colorful, luminous envelope of flamelike rays around the body. These images are certainly quite beautiful, but physicists remain highly skeptical as to their actual significance because of the great many parameters that come into play in the way they vary from one another.

However, there are a number of particularly interesting properties that prompt question. If you take an electro-photograph of a whole leaf, and then you cut the leaf into three pieces and take a second photo of the leaf in its thus mutilated state, you will see that a ghostlike image of the entire leaf will appear briefly with the image of cut leaf.

As with the vital field recorded in Burr's experiments, Kirlian photographs make it possible to view an energetic field to diagnose an individual's state of health as well as his or her emotional state.

The psychiatrist John Pierrakos, who pursued the ramifications of Burr's work in his own professional field, believes that the Kirlian phenomenon is only *a manifestation of Burr's electromagnetic field.* But the interaction between these two fields is still poorly understood.

The Russian scientist Victor Adamenko has shown that the acupuncture points and meridians of traditional Chinese medicine correspond to the most intensely colored and luminous points on a Kirlian photograph.

It just so happens that research pursued in France, in the department of physics and biophysics of the Pitié-Salpêtrière hospital, by Dr. Vernejoul, have shown that these points beneath the skin demonstrate a modest level of electrical resistance.

According to Régis Dutheil, we can thereby conclude the existence of a still poorly known structure that is entangled within the biological structure as opposed to overlaying it—something we could call the electrical body. There can be no doubt that this *body electric* will be at the very heart of future medicine and biology. This electrical body would therefore serve as an intermediary or mediator between consciousness and the body.

This electromagnetic field is concentrated in nodal points—it is possible to establish a very intriguing correspondence between this field and Hindu chakras or acupuncture points—that are primarily located in the area of the brain.

We now know that acupuncture points reveal a minimal amount of electrical resistance; in other words, they demonstrate maximal conductivity. We now know that human tissue possesses transistor properties, because it is able to transmit electrical current over a great distance.

So what can we establish concerning this electrical property of acupuncture points?

The flow of electrons circulating between the various acupuncture points could well be the famous energy cited by the Chinese—chi. Furthermore, the notions of yin and yang can be suggestive of a negative charge and a positive charge. It is thereby fairly obvious that if an entire electrical network is passing through these meridians, its local and overall intensity can be disrupted depending on the status of the health of the organ connected with a particular meridian.

We have to accept, and according to Régis Dutheil it is not such an extraordinary thing, that every organ has its own cutaneous electrical projection. Therefore, if we know that every organ without exception demonstrates electrical activity, it is perfectly plausible that this electrical body would simply be the topographical depiction of the different molecular structures that make up the body.

Any deficiency in the function of a given organ is going to produce a change in the electrical current this organ produces. By acting upon certain points in different ways (needles, massages), we change the organ's conductivity, which in turn has an effect upon its electrical activity.

This magnetic field notion has been known for a long time; Eastern traditions refer to it by a number of different terms, such as energy field or aura.

This is a topic that has been of great interest to me both personally and professionally. I have met different people who possessed the talent of seeing auras and used it as a basis for making diagnoses and reestablishing balance. Beyond the very real, concrete results I can vouch for personally, what really stands out for me is that everyone has their own way of seeing the aura.

To Recap

Three different levels exist within any living being:

- The molecular level that makes up the body
- The electrical level formed by the electromagnetic field
- The tachyonic plane corresponding to consciousness, which is the field of tachyonic matter and the headquarters of information (memory)

These three aspects are occupied by particles traveling at different speeds: slower than light on the molecular dimension and faster than light on the tachyonic level. Interactions in both directions are therefore continually taking place between the subluminous hologram (the *soma* or body), the electromagnetic body, and the tachyonic structure (consciousness).

The universe consists of two regions:

1. The physical region of everything that can be observed (this would be the ordinary reality as defined by Jean E. Charon, the subluminous realm of Régis Dutheil, Johann Soulas's "R.M." region, David Bohm's explicate order, and so on) using the basic senses of life (sight, touch, hearing) is essentially governed by time, energy, and entropy (everything that exists will inevitably become disorganized). This is the domain of matter and electromagnetic radiation. All material particles "travel" at infraluminous speeds (speeds that are slower than that of light).

2. The nonphysical region of the universe, meaning that which is immaterial and not observable by our physical senses. (This is the imaginal realm of Jean E. Charon, the superluminous one of Régis Dutheil, the "R.S." region of Johann Soulas, David Bohm's implicate order, Karl Pribam's frequency domain, Rupert Sheldrake's morphic field, and so forth.) This region is essentially governed by space. Time, as we conceive it, no longer exists.

This second region is governed by information and memory-based causality (memory saved in an indelible manner). This is the domain of immateriality, hence it is fundamentally the domain of the mind, of spirit. Here information can attain very high levels of organization. It is transported by nonmaterial particles known as tachyons, which are superluminous.

These tachyons produce a subtle electromagnetic radiation (its properties are symmetrically identical to those of visible electromagnetism), or, to put it in more scientific terminology, tachyomagnetism (fields of subtle radiation).

Johann Soulas notes that we have observed that all subtle forms of information are *interconnected*. In other words, the dominant spatial factor of this region creates the infinite tachyonic speed from one spot in the universe to another.

All of these subtle radiations are nonlocalized by definition (simultaneously in all places and all times, as seen from our "physical observatory"). They are undetectable by apparatuses with a "mineral"-based technology, in other words, the standard devices. On the other hand, a living and conscious (psycho-bio-computing) "device" known as a human being is capable of detecting and measuring these subtle waves.

Thousands of hours devoted to different areas of research and numerous experiments enabled the physicist Johann Soulas to show evidence of the infinite diversity of these radiations and to measure their properties. These fields would thereby be the original translation of spirit. These subtle measurements show that these radiation fields are responsible for the material "energetic condensation" within our temporal reference point (the visible universe). By virtue of this, all material substances, inert or not, are "induced" by one or more sources of subtle radiation, by nature similarly electromagnetic, which can explain, while remaining its originator, all evolution of matter. We call these sources, some of which were detected by the ancient civilizations of the East, subtle bodies, in accordance with those same ancient Eastern traditions (for more, see appendix 2).

Here is a very quick summary of Johann Soulas's theories. By means of its two radiant polarities, Consciousness (subtle electric nature) and Love (subtle magnetic nature), the (original) divine field gave birth to *four fields of subtle radiation:* spiritual, akashic, causal, and etheric. Those of the universe induce ten sources of highly informative subtle radiation (ten subtle bodies), which organize the life of the entire individual through his physical body:

- Lower etheric body
- Higher etheric body (*prana*)
- Lower astral body
- Middle astral body
- Higher astral body
- Lower mental body
- Higher mental body

These seven bodies constitute the "self" of every individual (his or her soul).

- The causal body—the body of all "good" and "bad" memories
- The akashic body (which could also be called the Christ body or the Buddha body)
- The spiritual body, which connects us directly to the sacred

These three other bodies constitute the individual's *transpersonal* aspect, what Kabbalists and Eastern mystics call the "self." They are made up of the countless frames of memory woven together over the course of the ages and the individual's connections with the sacred (or what we can still call the universe).

Note: I can only offer a bird's-eye view of this subject here. I am working on a future book that will examine our "energies" in depth.

We started with the chicken and the egg and took a long detour through the different landscapes of knowledge: that of everyday life observation, that of the traditions, that of the neurosciences, and that of relativistic quantum physics.

These different areas of research intersect with and enrich one another, and they are often quite akin. They make it possible to open our field of understanding, to open our mind about what and who we are, and allow us to know more concretely, more objectively, and more broadly the infinite relativity of things, thus acquainting us with all the infinite possibilities.

Our understanding and knowledge will therefore also be broader and more open, just as our hopes will be larger and wider . . . When we touch our bodies, the mind and energy are not far away!

Remember that in every cell of your body (with the brain forming part of the body), there is a dimension of spirit and energy. The skin you touch and the muscle you massage are a collection of cells, which themselves are made up of atoms primarily consisting of electromagnetic energy—electrons—one facet of which is providing a support material for the mind and the evolution of consciousness.

Like an orchestra, these cells form a collective entity while maintaining their individual distinctions (wind instruments, strings, and so on). Each plays its part of the score, and all play a part in the entire symphony.

When you touch your body, you are not only touching pure matter (which would not make any sense or be a scientific reality), you are also touching the mind, the packaging of the psyche (which includes sensations, emotions, feelings, and thoughts). In their own way, the sciences have objectively demonstrated this original continuum of the mind-body.

The body-mind duality would appear to be the chief distinguishing characteristic of human beings. It is due to their unique ability to dissociate themselves from their instincts, from their animal nature. Human beings not only have the ability to choose and to stand back; they also have the capacity to "sever" themselves from certain dimensions (sensorial, emotional, energetic) of their being.

4 • THE PROFOUND ONENESS OF BEING

You cannot pick a flower without disturbing a star.

CHINESE PROVERB

What we can take from all of this is that the human being is deeply, originally, phylogenetically,* ontologically, energetically, and neurologically unitary and synergistic in its functioning. Physics, neuroscience, personal observations, and traditions have, each in its own way, using its own words and experiences, all traveled in this same direction.

Every day my professional and personal practice confirms this a little more and lets me grasp a little more concretely the meaning of the saying "Everything is in everything."

One action (for example, pressing or sliding your hand over one part of the body) can cause an echo at a more distant location, either horizontally, between the different areas of the body, or vertically, "resonating" through feelings or emotions. Evidence for this appears to me every day in the performance of my practice.

This repercussion is going to depend on the individual's physical, emotional, and mental state, as well as his or her expectations, and the therapist's own state and intention. Everything happening between these parameters is the alchemy that allows a particular "inscription" at a given moment. Everything is potentially possible.

---

*Phylogenesis concerns the evolutionary history of a species, or of life since cells first appeared.

The Horizontal Level

There are numerous techniques in the domain of kinesitherapy, of corporeal synchronization, that rely upon the connections existing within a particular tissue layer (the muscles or the fasciae,* for example) and between several different layers of tissue (for example, the muscles, organs, skin, and fasciae).

I am now going to give you a few fairly common examples to help you grasp the nature of this "infinite entanglement."

Reflex Massage Techniques

These techniques include Dr. Henri Jarricot's reflex dermalgia (body-reflex therapy), *Bindegewebsmassage* (connective tissue massage—a whole-body massage), and reflexology of the foot, hands, and/or ears.

Here, every zone of the skin has a direct connection with a specific organ or body function. Each of these zones is therefore the means for diagnosing the problem and the spot where the therapist first applies stimulation.

The Notion of Chains

The significance of muscle chains is demonstrated by the manner in which the influence of one link in the chain has an effect on the remaining links (for example, how the tension in one muscle will be echoed by the other muscles in the chain connected to it).

This emphasis on muscle chains can be found in the postural reconstruction work of Françoise Mézières, Philippe Souchard's global postural reeducation (RPG), the "psychosomatic" chains of Godelieve Denys-Struyf, the "embryological" chains of microkinesis, the "beginning and end of chains" in myotherapy, Busquet's visceral, mechanical, and brain chains, and so forth.

I became very interested in these different approaches, particularly the work of Denys-Struyf (with its connection between the different mental components—biotypes—and how they are inscribed within the muscular-visceral-fascial patterns) and Busquet's theory on muscle chains, which is a magnificent work of synthesis (with a few variations on their muscular composition).

---

*Fasciae are sheets or bands of connective tissue that cover tissues and serve to separate or join different layers of tissue and enclose muscles, organs, and other soft structures of the body.

Each of these notions captures a multifaceted reality with multiple levels. It is the mystery of this incredible unity and complexity of the human being and the human body, the countless interactions between muscles or between muscles and the other tissues (skin, fasciae, organs . . .) through various mechanisms and reflexes, both energetic and embryological, as well as the role played therein by intention.

Some of these relationships have been codified and can be replicated by practitioners, but their mechanics cannot always be demonstrated scientifically. All the same, they work! The question remains: how and why?

Let's look at a small example: The number 1 point on the kidney, in energy medicine, is located at the same place as the point of the solar plexus in foot reflexology. Is it the intention that chooses which point is acted upon?

To better grasp the complexity of these interrelationships and this notion of holistic nature, I would like to linger for a moment over the importance of the psycho-emotional dimension, how it is encoded into the body, and the profound impact it has on our physical health.

The Vertical Level

Bodies and Emotions

Neuroscience has offered us clear and objective proof that *separating the mind from the body is pure absurdity* and utter nonsense, scientifically speaking.

Our emotions are only the conscious experience of a large set of *physiological reactions* that constantly supervise and are continuously adjusting our bodies' biological systems in response to internal and external imperatives. Our emotional experience is therefore constructed out of awareness of the changes taking place in our bodies, changes that can be neurological, muscular, circulatory, or biochemical in nature.

Every emotion, whether it is a basic one such as anger or sorrow or a social one such as sympathy, guilt, or shame, corresponds to a specific configuration of the body. *Physical changes therefore come before the emotional experience:* I am scared because I am trembling.

The origin of emotional life is physical, not verbal. We learn when things touch us. Emotional bonds, separation, feelings, and needs and their satisfaction are all first experienced through the body. The way in which, the reason why, and the time when someone sweeps us away or lets us down, embraces or rejects us, is going to determine the quality of our emotional life.

What we are learning at these times, for better or worse, is going to form the framework for our subsequent emotional life. It determines whether or not our behavior is appropriate in the relations we enjoy as children, adults, and parents and provides us with the personal resources we need to overcome the different challenges we shall face through life. What we assimilate at these times, what we "incorporate," is what we learn through our bodies.

As we can see, our bodies are the source of our emotions, but they are also the storehouse of our entire emotional life history (our personal memories, our cellular memories), which goes back quite far and for which we are the keepers. We inherit the history of the universe (specific memories going back some fifteen billion years), of life (phylogeny), of our family tree (psychogenealogy), of our forebears, of our intrauterine life (Stanislav Grof's perinatal matrixes), and of our own histories from birth to the present (biography).

Out of this legacy, there are a multitude of memories of negative and traumatizing experiences, memories of emotional shocks and conflicts that have not been digested and expelled, never expressed or resolved, memories that can no longer even be heard and of which we remain unaware but which always remain embedded within a cerebro-autonomic nervous-muscular network. They leave their negative traces on different levels (biological, physiological, mechanical, muscular, fascial, visceral), causing a sense of imbalance (blockage, tension, dysfunction, pain, and so forth).

Science itself now confirms this: the body itself is the best doctor for all our ills. It is the royal way to reach the emotions, as it is both their source and their storehouse.

Emotion and Its Corporeal Inscription
I have had the opportunity to work this emotional dimension through different disciplines and to approach others through reading. Some maintain that specific emotions are imprinted into specific zones of the body and establish tables of correspondence between certain emotions and certain sites of the body. The problem here is that each discipline does not always situate the same emotion at the same site, yet all these disciplines can show results.

The scientific understanding of the brain and the nervous system is already running up against the problem of a precise localization of emotions in the body. Furthermore, this notion—a place for every emotion and every emotion in its place—often restricts an individual's grasp of his or her own emotional experience.

My personal and clinical experience has shown me that any emotion can be connected to any part of the body, and that every part of the body can be linked to every emotion. Sometimes several emotions arise from the same part of the body, whereas at times several different threads connected to the same emotional experience can appear in different zones.

Each emotion corresponds to a configuration of the body and to neurological, muscular, circulatory, or biochemical changes. Looking at a sad individual, you will see that his physical expression of sorrow is global in nature (and that this physical expression has a stark difference from that of someone who is mad or happy). You shall see that these changes involve the entire body, from head to toe, and from the skin down into the bones and organs (see chapter 2).

This means that each zone of the body (vertebral axis, spinal column, waist, limbs, to mention only the dimension consisting of the joints and muscles) participates in an emotional expression in its own way, like the different instruments playing in an orchestra.

If an emotion expresses itself in "a configuration of the entire body," then this emotion can be contacted in any spot of this configuration. Grasping this fact can only enrich our approach and reduce our sectarian tendencies. An important spot then would be the one that the individual spontaneously indicates when asked to point to the physical zone that seems to be connected with the emotion, the place where it is felt most specifically.

The Notion of Armoring

Armor is the pure expression of an inhibited life. It displays imprisonment, inhibition, defense, and protection and is associated not with any specific muscles but with a network: muscle chains, bones, organs, blood, lymph, fasciae, interstitial fluids, and so on. It is connected not to one emotion but to a cluster of emotions, thoughts, images, and/or impressions commonly called the *affect*. It inscribes itself within the body unconsciously.

Wilhelm Reich, the father of corporeal psychology, was the first to talk about armoring. He believed that the expression of life and its movement were connected with universal energy. It circulated from top to bottom and vice versa in the form of vibratory waves that follow the longitudinal axis of the body. He discovered that his patients "wore" their inhibitions, which were inscribed into their bodies in the form of rings at different sections of the body. It was these rings that formed what he called character armor. His research allowed him to discover seven of these rings:

1. Ocular
2. Oral
3. Neck
4. Chest
5. Diaphragm
6. Abdomen
7. Pelvis

See appendix 3 for more about Reich's armoring.

Over the course of my professional life, I have had the opportunity to work with Marie-Lise Labonté, an individual who has made a deep inward journey to reach the heart of the body.* Over the years she studied its muscular and emotional expression in its own nonverbal language. In the beginning she relied on the grid established by Reich, but she then went on to expand and refine this notion of armoring, which she dubbed breastplates. Here is a quick summary of her discoveries.

As in an onion, the breastplates of identification make up the superficial layers of the skin, whereas the basic breastplates can be likened to the layers that surround the heart of the onion in order to protect it.

---

*The heart of our body is that physical area including the spinal column, its intrinsic muscles, and the central nervous system. This zone is in resonance with our true self, our true identity. In numerous traditions, this is also the place where the fundamental energy circulates. To learn more, read Labonté's book, *Au Coeur de notre corps* (Ed. de l'Homme, 2000).

Age	Type of Breastplate	The Corresponding Body
From 5 to 21 years	Breastplate of protection	Developed body
From 4 to 10 years	Breastplate of the poorly loved	Overridden body
From 2 to 7 years	Breastplate of despair	Ill body
From intrauterine life to 2 years	Fundamental breastplate	Body and poison of death

The Basic Breastplates

Fundamental breastplate

Breastplate of despair (impotence)

Breastplate of the poorly loved

Breastplate of protection

The heart of our body

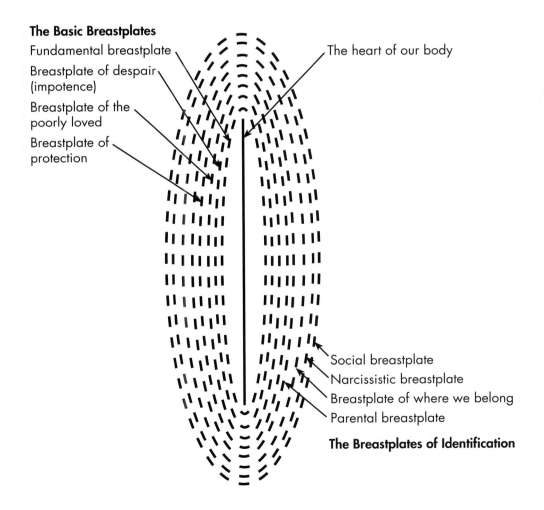

Social breastplate

Narcissistic breastplate

Breastplate of where we belong

Parental breastplate

The Breastplates of Identification

COMPARATIVE SUMMARY TABLE OF BREASTPLATES

The Breastplates of Identification

The breastplates of identification are the breastplates we put on during the quest for our identity through our parents, the other, clans, style, or society. They are connected with our parental and social history. They form part of the legend of our conditioning and the gilded cage in which we choose to live.

Age	Type of Breastplate	The Corresponding Body
30 years and older	Social breastplate	Conforming body
13 years and older	Narcissistic breastplate	"Beautiful" body
From 13 to 21	Breastplate of where we belong	Group body
From 5 to 18	Parental breastplate	Body of the parents

The Basic Breastplates

The basic breastplates are the breastplates that are built from the time of intrauterine life through adolescence and even later. These are the defense layers that are installed as a survival reaction to the different assaults, crises, and ordeals that form a natural part of life. They are connected to our deep history, and we are often unconscious of their existence. This is what we call the key to our personal legend, that which makes each of us a unique individual different from other people. This personal legend belongs to us alone, and once it has been grasped, heard, and understood, it will suddenly provide a meaning to our lives.

To Recap

Let's look at the simple example of a pulled and painful muscle:

- It could be the result of an involuntary contraction, direct assault (something struck it), excessive work, violent stretching, a surgical operation, and so on.
- It could be suffering repercussions from other muscles (in mechanical or embryological chains) as a result of reflex or analgesic interactions.

- It could be the influence of the disruption of another tissue: skin, viscera, fasciae.
- Because it is a part of the body-mind continuum, it reflects the emotional and mental state of the individual (and is in any case inscribed within the cerebral neuromuscular patterns).
- It could be the point targeted by the brain's "survival programming" (see chapter 8).

These different vertical and horizontal levels are inscribed in our muscles at every instant. Consequently, a technique that is active on a particular level can have spectacular results, for example, eliminating a pain by removing a factor from the persona that was greatly contributing to it. Another individual, after hearing how great this technique is, may turn to it full of hope and be greatly disappointed. The reason is that the factor this technique treats so effectively was of less influence in the second person's mind-body makeup.

We should look at all these techniques, even those that are all the rage, as simply being another piece of the puzzle.

Note: And we should not come to the conclusion that because the pain is gone the zone is now truly relaxed. It could still be like a vase ready to overflow!

Imagine an acupuncture session to balance the energies, a massage for relaxation, a reflexology session to work on a particular organ or function, taking a dietary supplement, and so forth. These actions all possess true intrinsic value and all play a role in establishing balance in the different elements of our health. We should not take them as recipes so much as view them as ways to get the ball rolling, so to speak, or better yet the wheel. They are helpful in maintaining (not creating) the movement of the wheel of our health and balance. They should be integrated into a holistic approach offering an overall understanding.

Let's not forget that we "function" in deep unity and synergy. Let's open our minds and trust our ability to heal ourselves, to soundly implement a life dynamic that goes well beyond our learning and intelligence. This is a fundamental energy, a self-regulating force, and a life intelligence. It does not matter what words we choose to talk about this thing that animates us and the life that has made us "so intelligent." In any case, it must surely be more intelligent! Place your trust in it and give it a little nudge.

The doctor treats wounds, God cures them.
HIPPOCRATES

The human being is always functioning on the different levels (vertical and horizontal) simultaneously. By touching the body, I am able to reach these levels, but my reach depends in large part on my intention, my approach, my ability to tune in, and my awareness (and that of the patient, of course).

5 • INTENTION

The word *intention* comes from the Latin *intentus,* which, literally translated, means "unfolding outward" or "unfolding toward." Although it is hard to identify, intention is an important part of the therapeutic exchange. It presupposes the goodwill of the accompanying and the accompanied individual: their conscious and unconscious hopes, their expectations, and their individual needs.

Here are several studies that demonstrate the power of a conscious intention and its importance in a therapeutic exchange.

During the 1990s, a research project was undertaken by Canada's National Institute of Mental Health to determine the effectiveness of psychotherapy. Patients were randomly sent to qualified and unqualified therapists, not knowing which they would be seeing.

The unqualified therapists had been taught a technique of empathic listening. They simply possessed the intention of looking at their patients with the greatest consideration and kindly listening to them without adding any analysis or additional commentary.

The progress of the two groups was measured at regular intervals. After six months there were no noticeable differences between the patients of the two groups. This study made it possible to conclude that the attitude or intention of the therapist toward his or her patient was an essential ingredient of effective therapy.

In the beginning, intention by itself was sufficient to provide positive results.

A complementary study made it possible to examine patients' reaction to therapeutic intention. Joseph Weiss and his colleagues tested two hypotheses concerning the way people in therapy changed:

- The first suggests that the therapist tests the patient's readiness to change.
- The second suggests that the client tests the therapist's readiness for the patient to change.

At the conclusion of a long series of tests, Weiss was led to support the second hypothesis.

Although these studies speak volumes about the importance of intention in therapy-generated change, they say little about the way in which intention truly allows that change to occur.

Several scientific studies also suggest that the power of intention can have an influence on animate and inanimate objects. Carroll Nash, a biologist at Saint Joseph's University in Philadelphia, studied the effects of intention on the genetic mutation of bacteria. In one study, he used *Escherichia coli,* which normally undergoes mutation from one type to another at a predictable rate. Fifty-two people were asked to concentrate on either encouraging or hampering this mutation. With the *E. coli* in nine test tubes, volunteers were asked to focus their intention on hindering the mutation in three test tubes and on encouraging the mutation in three others. The remaining three test tubes served as controls for the experiment.

The results were very significant.

J. Williams and his colleagues performed a series of experiments on human subjects at the Mind Science Foundation.* They connected electrodes to the palms and fingers of the experiment subjects to measure the electrical activity of their skin. Other groups of volunteers, placed in separate rooms, were asked to influence the electrical activity of the skin of the subjects in the first group. They succeeded, even when subjects in the first group were not aware of their participation!

Other experiments, notably those involving the formation of water crystals, provided evidence of the very specific influence of intention upon matter. (There was a time when I found great amusement in "mummifying" steaks through the "magnetic" effect of my hands. I have kept a sample of one in a drawer for now more than thirty years.)

Even if this appears to entirely counter to common sense, *the intention of an individual acts on the body and the mind of another person.*

---

*As reported in *Brain/Mind Bulletin* no. 9 (1984).

The EPR Paradox

Although these experiments may be amazing and significant, they do not always offer an explanation for how intention can produce effects like these. We have been able to establish a somewhat more tangible hypothesis thanks to the doubts voiced by the great scientist Albert Einstein.

The central figure in a far-ranging debate on how best to describe reality, Einstein was one of a group of relativists who suggested a commonsense approach to this question. They believed reality could best be described on the basis of observations and measurements.

But quantum theory was in complete opposition to this idea! Reality, to the quantum theoreticians, could not be measured or observed with any exactitude, and therefore it would be impossible to describe except through tendencies or probabilities. "God does not play dice," was Einstein's famous retort.

In the 1930s Einstein and two of his colleagues, Boris Podolsky and Nathan Rosen, proposed the following absurd assertion that would have to be correct if quantum theory was right: Take two particles belonging to the same system, which are entangled in such a way as to make them identical. Send each of them to opposite ends of the universe, and then change the trajectory of one of them. The trajectory of the other would then also change—instantaneously. The theory that the change of one particle's trajectory had caused the other's to change would be automatically ruled out, because according to quantum theory, the two trajectories would change simultaneously.

An experimental facility was then devised. Two particles would be separated inside a research laboratory to such a distance from each other that no known physical force could be operated upon one by the other. The change of the one particle's trajectory could therefore not be responsible for or cause that of the other. The rotation of one of the particles was then altered and—instantly—that of the other changed. To the great surprise of many scientists, the paradox turned out to be right!

What does the EPR (Einstein Podolsky Rosen) paradox teach us about intention? It tells us that events occur within an order of reality based on unity and not on separation. Any change in one point of the universe alters all the conditions in the universe. This is known as the butterfly effect.

Intention is therefore able to act in this order of reality. The particles described in the EPR paradox do not need to be photons or electrons isolated in an experimental apparatus in a research lab. Everything takes place as if each point of the universe instantaneously "knows" what is happening in another point and reacts to it.

Every time one human being touches another human being, the conditions of the EPR paradox come into play. Even if you do not touch someone but simply stand close to him or her, a particle exchange takes place. Now, if you leave your partner for a time and something changes inside of you, according to the EPR paradox, a change will occur simultaneously in him or her.

A feeling or a thought directed toward someone else is enough to produce this change simultaneously in that person. It yet remains to be seen if intention will one day be demonstrable in the terms of quantum physics!

In my practice of conscious touch, I am able to verify the importance and influence of the conscious and directed dimension of intention. Here are a few memorable experiments I often suggest to the people taking my workshops on touch. They are excellent illustrations of the arguments I am making in this book.

1. Lightly touch someone. Without changing the intensity, duration, or direction of this contact, simply focus on transmitting your intention. The person on the receiving end of this contact will try to feel what quality has been intentionally put forth: love, hate, fear, guilt . . . Many participants are able to sense this change of intent and to correctly feel what was intentionally put forth.

2. Rest your hands on either side of your partner's shoulder and very slowly slide them down the length of his or her arm to the fingers, scrupulously following the shape of the limb. Do this several times:

   - Once while thinking of a neutral topic like the weather (not focusing attention on your partner)
   - Then with the intention of fully sensing the surface and volume of the arm
   - Then with the intention of connecting with the energetic dimension and distributing this energy into the arm equally
   - Finally with the intention of emptying the arm of its energy

Note: Of course, the partners are not told of these intentions.

If two partners play the game and are receptive and clear in their intention, I promise you that they will clearly feel the differences among these four intentions and that they will not have the "same arm."

If the notion of energy fails to speak to you, if you don't really believe in it, if you really do not grasp what needs to be done and just go through the motions, the result will be not at all convincing, especially if your partner is equally as skeptical, does not want to try this experiment, or has failed to understand its purpose.

For the receiver, the difference between an intention based in skepticism and an intention based in full belief and comprehension is extremely clear-cut.

Intention is a little like the hand that turns the dial on a radio, trying to tune in to a particular station. Potentially speaking, all stations are present, but in the reality of the radio set, the choice is limited. The same is true for the individual.

We are ontologically restricted, even if our intention is to have no intention, to open up completely. My constitution, my education and professional training, my beliefs, and my emotional and psychological blocks all ensure that my opening is conditioned and oriented in a particular direction. Life can only apprehend itself through the small end of the telescope, even if that view piece can be enlarged.

I would like to illustrate this contention with several examples. If I ask several different people to place their hands in the same way on a person's head and tune in to his skull and allow the sensations to just flow in, each person is going to feel things a little differently:

- The trained osteopath is going to spontaneously detect certain cranial movements in particular.
- The energy or faith healer will detect energy currents and the properties of different energies while entirely overlooking cranial movement.
- An individual who is very intuitive and highly sensitive will see colors or images, or feel emotions.
- Personally, what I am most aware of when performing this experiment is something that I define as the feeling of a certain state, a level of life that inhabits the tissues.

In front of me there is a small path. There is a large tree some twenty or thirty yards away, next to which a river is flowing. On the other side of the river, far away, I can see bushes. I am confident in my description, which is of the reality before my eyes.

Another person, who is directly opposite my position, sees a lot of bushes and a little farther away the flowing river. In the background she can see a path with a large tree next to it. She, too, is sure she is being entirely objective.

A third person walking in the middle of the stream has the brief impression that the other two people are totally mistaken: first there is the river, and then, further away, are bushes on one bank and a path on the other.

For me the river comes after the path; for the person on the other side of the river the reverse is obviously true. And the third person thinks both of us are wrong. I am not even mentioning the person in the hot-air balloon, who sees the landscape completely differently and would not recognize the description given by the others as being of the same countryside. While what each is saying is correct, their points of view and their apprehension are different.

By virtue of their individual histories, how open-minded they are, their conditioning, their education, and their beliefs, each one of these individuals catches the landscape from a certain angle.

In the health field there currently exists such a wide variety of corporeal approaches that it is quite difficult to find your way around and make an intelligent choice. Many seem to be in conflict or diametrically opposed to others. One person says white; another says black. Remember what we just learned about the notion of "objective" perspective: white may be just as true as black, or indeed red (see appendix 4).

Every individual's perception serves as a working context: each has its value and effectiveness, as well as, of course, its limitations. The experience of different points of view helps us to better situate ourselves and to be less sectarian. It opens for us doors of action, understanding, hope, and increased potential for health and well-being.

To Recap

Intention provides awareness with a certain direction. It allows us to connect, to "select" a certain aspect of the present reality, of this mind-body continuum, even if we are not aware of it.

Consciousness is the feeling, the lived experience, and what we perceive of reality.

The directions taken by this intention are infinite, just like the interrelations between reality's various aspects, but the intention is limited. First and foremost, it is limited by the fact that if I do not believe something is possible or am completely unaware that it even exists, I can form no intention concerning it. It is next limited by the fact that if the intention is there but I really do not understand it, I am unable to really believe in it, or I harbor doubts about it, then a real connection cannot be made.

6 • TOTAL HEALTH

When someone falls ill, it is necessary to change his way of living,
because no healing can take place without a mental and spiritual
effort.

HIPPOCRATES

Illness is the effort Nature makes to heal us.

CARL GUSTAV JUNG

What is health?

Let's start by examining the definition offered by the World Health Organization: "Health is a state of complete physical, mental, and social well-being and not merely the absence of disease or infirmity."

Are we in good health?

This definition brings to mind holistic approaches that define health as the result of the harmonious balance of all the individual's component parts, his environment, and, in an even broader sense, the entire universe.

As I said earlier, our state of health is a question of a global nature. The mental and emotional dimensions are not separate from the physical matter of which we are made; other aspects of our life influence the state of our physiological health.

Neurologically, energetically, and scientifically speaking, your physical state is also your mental and emotional state. This is why when some people hear a healthcare practitioner tell them, "It's psychological!" or "It's all in your head!" or "There's nothing wrong with you, all your tests came back negative!" they wonder if they are "going crazy." I have always been astounded (and I am being diplomatic when

I use that word!) by responses like these and this kind of reasoning, which is at the antipodes of that science for which these practitioners are allegedly the best representatives.

As you may well imagine, equilibrium is not a state that is acquired once and for all. Rather, it requires constant efforts to maintain and stabilize (like keeping your balance on a bicycle). This balanced state of health is particularly difficult to maintain now thanks to the increasing number of disruptive factors, for example the pollutants that we come into contact with, ingest, and breathe from morning to night.

It is getting harder and harder for us to "assimilate" and to "digest." It is imperative that we make time for ourselves, in one way or another, to rest, to let our orthosympathetic* system do its job, to calm our mind, to be in a state of nonaction, which will thereby allow our potential to establish homeostasis to manifest. These processes are not abstract ideas or simply words but concrete manifestations that I encounter in my work and around me.

How deeply ungrateful we are to life; what ingrates we are toward this intelligence that is the source of all our creations, that does everything to keep us alive and help us restore our balance, sometimes even to the point of helping us to feel the exhaustion, at which point the symptoms are often mistaken for the cause. There is no such thing as a pill, massage, technique, or miracle potion that will give you health on a platter without your personal participation and involvement.

This true, profound health of the body is also a matter that involves the heart, the mind, and consciousness.

Healing, Illness, Symptoms, Self-Healing

What is illness; what is healing? These questions appear so simple at first glance that many people no longer even ask them, and yet . . . !

The purpose of this chapter is not to deal with this vast subject, which has already been the subject of thousands of books, in any exhaustive fashion but simply to bring up a few ideas for consideration.

The word *healing* is most often associated with the disappearance of a symptom or an illness. The problem (which you can verify for yourself in many cases)

---

*The orthosympathetic system is a part of the autonomic nervous system that functions when we are active, under stress, and so on.

is that eliminating the symptom does not equate with removing the cause: you are simply driving it away, and it often returns at top speed—and not always by the same path!

What is a symptom? What is it a manifestation of? What does it mean?

- If we systematically look at symptoms (acne, fever, diarrhea, and so on) as the expression of an illness, our efforts are going to be focused on eliminating the illness, no matter what the cost.
- If the displayed symptoms are understood as part of a larger, more global process and not necessarily a negative one, our systematic compulsion will be not to remove them but to lessen them, in order to restore balance to the terrain (the internal cellular environment), as in homeopathy or naturopathy, or to restore balance to our energy, as in acupuncture and other energy-point therapies.
- Now, if we envision certain symptoms as being not part of a process throwing things out of balance but as manifestations of the body's attempt to restore homeostasis, that viewpoint will change many things in the way we intervene therapeutically.

This may appear to be pure nonsense and completely loony, yet this is how it works all the same. I am not going to explore this concept in great detail—this is not the purpose of this book. I am not asking you to take me at my word, though; I am simply inviting you to become better informed through study and practice, and your own observations, and basically to get off the beaten path.

This expanded viewpoint offers great hope for our understanding of a large number of diseases, but it also poses a challenge to the status quo and many vested interests. Falling out of balance is a process through which pathological conditions that are conducive to illness become established in a way that is both silent and painless. The process of restoring balance to the body, or homeostasis, is quite often more noticeable, and its symptoms are often much more evident. We may feel worse, our fevers may run higher, we may have more acne, we are often more tired—the list can go on and on.

We often then think that we are sick, and the actions we take to address sickness consequently serve to block the healing process (of course, when symptoms are severe, it is often necessary to intervene to mitigate them). This understanding or confusion between a state of disequilibrium and one that is restoring balance will have consequences even for those people who are seeking to cure themselves by means of homeopathy, acupuncture, or other so-called alternative or holistic therapies.

I would like to illustrate this topic with some cases from my own practice and daily life.

Women in their fifties often come to see me complaining that they are always feeling tired and have no energy:

"I don't understand," they say to me. "I am in a period of my life where my children have all left the nest and I no longer have any responsibilities for them. I finally have time for me, all my health exams are good, and yet . . . !"

How should this be interpreted? What actions should they take? Should these patients take tonics, stimulants, or other powerful means to restore energy? This is often what most people do as they focus all their attention on eliminating the symptoms.

This is how I answer them:

"For twenty or thirty years you have had to work, manage the household, and raise your children without ever really taking the time you need to rest. Over these long months and years you have thereby accumulated fatigue, tensions, and stress that all your vacations and weekends could not really provide enough time to digest thoroughly. Now that you have reached a period of your life that is calmer both physically and psychologically, you are allowing your body, your life, to empty itself of all that. If you can understand what you are going through this way, you can accept this fatigue and give your body a helping hand to facilitate this clearing and everything will return to order. But this will not happen in two weeks; it will take several months."

And this is what did happen gradually over the succeeding therapy sessions, after which these women were amazed to find themselves relaxed and full of energy.

This same phenomenon can be seen at the beginning of a vacation. You yourself may have been dismayed to find yourself exhausted and lacking all energy, with no desire to do anything: "I am having a hard time figuring this out. When I'm working I have energy, and when I'm not working I feel exhausted!"

Common sense would say here, too, that vacations are really times for recuperation and cleansing, without forgetting to have a good time. But because we have to take full advantage of this short time of freedom, often we use up this time in a way that is abusive to our health, and when we resume work, we feel all right mentally but not so fine physiologically and physically.

After a reharmonization session using any appropriate technique, there can often be an exacerbation of the symptoms on the following day. This will last from several hours to an entire day, if not longer, and then vanishes, giving way to a sense of feeling better when compared to before the session.

Sometimes treatment provides an opportunity for old symptoms to reappear: "It's funny, it is that very place where I first started to hurt a long time ago!" Here, too, is a mechanism that is restoring order, "unknotting tensions," and not something that is getting worse.

Countless other concrete examples exist concerning a wide variety of disorders. I can only repeat here my earlier invitation: open your mind and take the time to learn more about this subject; abandon the well-beaten paths that fear, ignorance, and disinformation maintain.

The truth is much vaster than you might think, albeit relative of course, but full of hope and potential.

7 • BIOHARMONY

Embodying the Self with Consciousness

How to meet yourself,
taking the path of the body

The unconsciousness of matter is a veiled, somnambulistic, imprisoned consciousness, which contains all the latent powers of Spirit.

In every particle, every atom, every molecule, every cell of matter, lives and labors, unknown, all the omniscience of the Eternal and all the omnipotence of the Infinite.

THE MOTHER'S AGENDA

Embodiment

It is through our corporeality that we apprehend the world and are able to feel, to think, and to be moved emotionally—or, to put it more simply, to live. Our entire personal history (our stress, traumas, various conflicts that remain poorly worked out or unexpressed) is inscribed within our body and incarnates there in the form of tensions in the tissue, states of energetic stasis, pains, psychosomatic symptoms, and an impoverishment of our sensations and corporeal awareness.

In the bioharmonic approach, our body is perceived and grasped not simply as a reflex zone, an energetic point requiring stimulation, a dysfunction that needs to be made to function properly, or a support for freeing emotions, but as a book that can be opened and can tell the story of our lives, our entire personal and relational history. This approach addresses simultaneously our physical bodies and our lived experience. The purpose of this work is to build awareness, the consequence of which is harmony.

Intention, Attitude, and State of Mind

My years of study and practice in a variety of touch therapies and massage (circulatory, energetic, reflex zone, emotional, eutonic, and so forth) led me to develop a kind of bodywork, and in particular a form of massage, whose intention is to welcome life (sensations, emotions, memories, energies, and so on), as it happens in the present, through the body and tissues that both embody it and express it.

I put myself in an attitude of nondoing, without any intention of applying any kind of beneficial action upon the body, whether it involves the relaxation of a tension, the soothing of a pain, or the expression of an emotion. The hand—in massage and therapy—and the other tools (self-massages, postures, and so on) offer patients the opportunity to connect with themselves through sensations, emotions, feelings, and interior images.

There is no adversary to be bested on this path, no foe to master, nothing to be eliminated (tensions, pains, and so forth). I operate inside a dynamic not of duality but of unification, of oneness.

I reach out to this attitude of receptivity and compassion, which is the key to real change, liberation, and oneness with the other. Compassion is often defined as empathy or sympathy that an individual can feel for the sufferings of another, while strongly wishing for their resolution. In fact, the word *compassion* comes from two Latin words: *com,* which means unity, cohesion, or togetherness, and *passion,* which means suffering. For this reason, a standard interpretation of *compassion* is "to suffer together." But *together* also means to become one with: to be one with someone's pain or tension. This is the opposite of denial. You are not ignoring it, and you are not attempting to resist it; you enter it deeply, through sensations, emotions, and feelings.

This compassionate approach using touch possesses a great deal of similarity to the positive and unconditional approach of Carl Rogers. These two expressions reflect an attitude of acceptance toward the accompanying person. This attitude encompasses the desire to allow the other person to display all feelings as they arise in the moment, with no thought of directing or influencing this individual.

Relaxation, harmony, and letting go are all expressive of an opening awareness, of the ability to become one with something. This awareness is able to function because of the existence of bioharmonic potentialities.

Wherever consciousness can establish itself, harmony can make itself at home.

Bioharmonic Therapy

This therapy relies primarily upon manual techniques (staying still, sliding, applying pressure, mini stretches, vibrations, and so on) that make it possible to contact the various levels and parts of the body (skin, fasciae, muscles, bones, organs, the circulatory system, the bioenergetic field).

In a state of shared receptive consciousness, the therapist and the patient will be simple catalysts of life movement and the inner dynamic of growth whose natural tendency is toward harmony.

These bioharmonic processes manifest on the physical level, particularly through an autonomic process (activation of the parasympathetic nervous system) of "physical and emotional digestion," which can be tangibly perceived by listening to the different sounds made by intestinal peristalsis with a stethoscope. This intestinal peristalsis is equivalent to the abdominal brain of the Chinese or the psychoperistalsis of G. Boyeson. This work often relies upon these auditory responses that facilitate letting go (the biofeedback principle) and thereby permit a structuring and balancing practice.

Every session is an excursion through the space of the self, during which I accompany the participating individual with conscious touch:

- I can remain silent and let the other individual spontaneously open up to his or her sensations and feelings, completely free to put them into words or to release an emotion while remaining connected to the here and now of the sensations.
- I can guide the individual through the "excursion" to help him or her obtain a deeper perception of certain aspects of the "countryside."
- I can, if the other person requests it, guide this stroll in an emotional direction.

Not only a path to self-knowledge, a path to restoring overall balance, and a profound technique for relaxation, bioharmony also possesses applications that are very practical in kinesiotherapy, including:

- In the domain of joint and muscle pain
- In stress management and sleep problems
- In psychosomatic disorders
- In postural reeducation

Bioharmony is complementary to the traditional verbal psychotherapy and can facilitate recognition and full integration of traumatic events through the release of the emotional charge that has been "scripted" into the body.

This approach invites us to find oneness, to "embody" ourselves in our consciousness by becoming open and receptive to our sensorial and spatial dimensions. Remember, this body made of skin and bones, muscles and organs, is essentially and fundamentally the source/expression of life in its sensorial, emotional, affective, mental, and spiritual dimensions.

I invite you to practice these massage techniques on yourself in this kind of open-mindedness and receptive consciousness.

In Concrete Terms

When you touch your body, the depth and extent of the result will be the fruit of the intention you put into it, which is connected to how well you comprehend yourself, as well as your understanding of your body, how you function, and what you think or believe you are able to do or what you think or believe is possible.

These self-massages call for the use of simple tools, which I call our true friends or mirror tools. They accompany us without making any judgments and reveal who we are to ourselves. They help us make contact with the state of life in the zone we are touching. Intention, pressure, speed, rhythm, the tool used, and each action on our body, our self, opens us to sensations. They make us receptive to a unique kind of feeling, one that invites us to be present in the moment and to welcome it.

8 • THE DIMENSIONS OF THE BODY

The mind is incidental to organic evolution from its very first stages and throughout the entire development of the animal kingdom. It is born with matter and transforms with it, until it becomes thought and consciousness.

GUY LAZORTHES

My purpose in this chapter is to provide you with a detailed explanation of the dimensions of the body, in particular the symbolic dimension. There are extremely good books in this field already. I would like to bring my own clarifications, through the contributions of the neurosciences, physics, phylogeny, embryology, and animal ethology, to help us better understand this dimension and put it into practice. So in order to better understand the overlapping of these different dimensions, I am inviting you to dive deep into the remote past with me.

First Stage

Several billion years ago life first made its appearance on this planet in the form of cells, very simple single-celled organisms that, in order to live and perpetuate as a species, had to breathe, eat, eliminate, and reproduce.

Over the passing of time, cells began to combine with other cells in order to adapt to and survive in a hostile environment. This was the advent of multi-cellular organisms. For example, if an organism inhabited an environment with scarce oxygen, it entered into a stress phase and eventually resolved the dilemma by multiplying the number of cells at its disposal for breathing. Through cellular proliferation—multiplying the cells it specifically needed for breathing, eating, eliminating, or reproducing—it ensured its survival through this stage. The command for this proliferation was generated by an archaic cerebral structure that was destined to become our brain stem.

Second Stage

The transition of living organisms from an aquatic environment to dry land took place during this period. Having resolved their basic survival issues, multicellular organisms still continued refining and perfecting themselves to protect themselves from the world around them. If, for example, they found the rays of the sun too aggressive, they caused their membranes to thicken in order to avoid being mortally stricken with sunburn.

Third Stage

During this stage life continued its evolution toward a more autonomous and conscious existence. This was the time in which the now more complex life-forms set off in exploration of the four corners of their terrestrial environment and confronted the outside world.

Life-forms thereby developed skeletons, muscles, and tendons that could give them additional support and allow for more effective movement that was better adapted to their surroundings. They formed a kind of bridge connecting the organs strictly necessary for maintaining life to those organs that were receptive to the outside world (for example, the sense organs), in the most general sense of the world.

But if this new world revealed an overly hostile aspect, life would reverse course and return to more familiar terrain, while more or less keeping, depending on circumstances, one foot in these new surroundings. This process would eliminate or shrink, again depending on the situation, the organs that had developed. With certain structures now stripped of any usefulness, the organism would have to undergo a period of cellular reduction or necrosis.

Fourth Stage

The fourth stage would host the consolidation of all the preceding stages. A transition was made from "I am moving on solid ground and I am testing myself in these new surroundings" to "I am establishing communication with other beings." The sensory organs and the conduits of liaison between the various organs were refined and perfected even further (the membranous tissue covering the organs and other internal body surfaces was formed now), as were the nervous system and motor nerves, making it possible for humans to establish relations with other human beings and society, in accordance with all the psychological subtleties this domain requires.

Life, in order to grow and perfect itself, and to become conscious of itself, had to overcome various obstacles in its path by making adaptations (cell proliferation, thickened membranes, autolysis, and so forth) and initiating biological survival programs, all implemented and committed to memory in extremely archaic cerebral structures (first stage), in order to reach the latest stage, that of the cerebral cortex.

These survival programs affected different aspects of life at each of these stages, but each successive stage held those of the previous stages in its memory, inscribed within corresponding nerve structures. We have therefore inherited from all the living things that preceded us the quintessence of these biological processes of adaptation and biodiversification.

We can see a parallel between this history of the development of the species over the course of evolution (phylogeny) and the process that unfolds in the maternal womb (embryogenesis), which recapitulates in some way all the stages of evolution, with the fetus resembling in turn an amoeba, a tadpole, and so on. During the first two months of its life, the fetus incarnates all these memories that span the long period between the origin of life and the present.

As the neurosciences have demonstrated, the brain is the conductor of this orchestra of our psychology. Every function and every part of our body is connected to a part of our brain. According to the data harvested in the most recent studies of neurophysiology, our brains should be regarded more as supercomputers, super organs for information processing, than as entities that think independently and are provided with discernment and reflexive awareness.

The brain treats all information in the same manner; it does not make any distinction between real or virtual, the symbolic or the imaginary. It is only consciousness that allows us to make such distinctions. Think of a very tart lemon wedge. Now imagine that you are biting right into it and its acidic juices are spilling over your tongue. What happens next? You will secrete more saliva. The brain gives commands in order to facilitate the digestion of this juice that does not really exist.

We need to realize that the brain makes no distinction between the real (the rabbit's foot stuck in the wolf's stomach) and the imaginary or symbolic (Paul is laid off and experiences this setback like a lead weight in his stomach). In the case of the wolf, the brain springs into action, commanding the triggering of a cellular proliferation (a superprogram for use in exceptional situations) of high-performance digestive supercells, which will allow the animal to survive. In Paul's case, things are a bit more complicated. The survival program is not triggered automatically; certain parameters are required. But if the factors are present, the digestive function (particularly the stomach) will be targeted.

What traces of these different evolutionary stages remain inscribed inside the brain of the modern human being? What conflictive events can cause their reemergence? I will briefly recap them below, though I cannot linger over it in great detail, as that would extend far beyond the scope of this book.

Stage 1: This involves conflicts concerning pieces (a mouthful of food, a gulp of air, and so forth) in the sense of not being able to get your teeth into it, not being able to swallow it, not being able to digest and eliminate it.

The idea of the mouthful can be experienced in its literal sense (I have nothing to eat), the figurative sense (my means of support has been cut because I lost a job, got divorced, and so on), or in an even more symbolic sense (I was turned down for a loan or an inheritance, or job that I was confident was in the bag fizzled out at the last moment, and so forth).

Stage 2: Generally speaking, these are conflicts connected with our own space, our frontiers (such as the skin that separates self from what is not self), linked with the fear of being attacked, suffering an assault against our physical identity or our physical integrity, a cruel assault on our moral integrity, a sense of being tainted or soiled.

Stage 3: Here it is necessary to confront an external world. The very individual problem of self-evaluation arises here. These conflicts involve self-depreciation, no longer feeling equal to the task, no longer feeling capable of finding satisfaction, no longer capable of having children or providing for them, and so forth.

Stage 4: The drama moves to the mental plane, where we witness projection of the self into an ever larger and more complex and changing context. It becomes increasingly difficult for us to ignore what is going on around us and not take into account the multiple situations that are characteristic of life.

Conflicts related to this stage involve the feeling that we are incapable of taking any quick action. There is also a sense of urgency, of danger, of being sick, of being panicked at the thought of death. These are also territorial conflicts and those caused by separation anxiety.

Returning to the various dimensions of the body and its symbology, the body was, phylogenetically speaking, first and foremost biological during an extremely long period, expressed through basic vital functions: reproduction, eating, elimination, breathing . . . Life was sensitive; this was the world of primary sensations, similar to that of the single-celled and then multicellular organisms. As time passed, life became more complex, evolving toward greater autonomy and consciousness. Sensations became more varied and subtle, taking us from the world of primary emotions and instincts to that of more complex and social emotions. Biological matter became imbued with the sensorial and the emotional.

Starting with stage 4 (which is quite recent when compared to the other stages), things picked up speed and became even more complicated, with the individual's newfound ability of self-awareness and capacity to disconnect from animal depths (it may be more correct to say biological depths) and understand, bestow meaning, contemplate, and project. This is the stage when mind appears, with thought, contemplation, and all its virtual, imaginary, and symbolic aspects (the human being is the youngest of life's children). Biological, sensorial, and emotional matter has become imbued with meaning, an imaginal realm, and a symbology.

Now humankind is seeking to explain and give meaning to all these aspects of reality. Depending on geography, era, and individual history, we form a point of view. Each is but a clarification and interpretation of deeply anchored beliefs.

They are so deeply rooted because they have been handed down and inherited as a fundamental truth, which thereby connects matter and the body, profoundly and unconsciously, with a meaning.

I believe that all this gives us a conditioned sense, one that conditions us in our functioning on every level, much more deeply and strongly than we imagine, and that is restrictive in this sense. Reconnecting with symbols and studying this symbology also means reestablishing contact with and being receptive to conditioning, and thus liberating potentials for finding harmony.

As far as how this concerns my practice of self-massages, its chief target is in the dimension of joints and muscles.

We need to realize that this massage system fundamentally enables us to concretely establish relations with the outside world, explore our environment, and set off on a journey through the four corners of the earth, doing, acting, expressing, and taking our own measure in this new world.

Where human beings are concerned, it is the development of our own value that is at stake, to the extent that we are going to have to confront the outside world here. The problem will be therefore one of self-evaluation, inasmuch as if the values we use as benchmarks should prove to be too heavy, we will feel diminished and not equal to the task, condemned to keep a low profile.

What we find here are conflicts of self-depreciation and the reduction of an individual's personal value in all its various shades (being unequal to, not being up to snuff, no longer mattering to anyone, feeling worthless or not as good as anyone else, feeling impotent, and so forth). Depending on just how this sense of self-devaluation expresses itself, a specific element of the joint and muscle system will be affected (bone, cartilage, muscle, tendon, ligament, periosteum, connective tissue, and so on). For that given element (the joints or muscles, for example), its involvement in the situation and how it is brought into play (for example, some muscles are used to repel and push away, to move away from other people, whereas other muscles are used to draw people in) will also be affected.

I am going to give a simple example. Let's imagine we are picking an apple from a tree. We will head toward this tree to get close enough to pick this fruit. It is our lower limbs that allow us to move toward that tree and take position, by moving a step forward or back, standing up on tiptoe, balancing on one leg, and so forth.

Each segment of the lower limbs (hips, thighs, knees, calves, ankles, feet) takes part in the realization of the most refined, adapted and adaptable, economical, and efficient movement possible. If you imagine that your hips are fixed in place, or that your knees or ankles are unable to bend or even move, you will be able to see the importance, the specificity, and the complementary nature of each part.

Physical problems affecting our lower limbs can express the fact that we are facing an attitude or role that makes it difficult for us to position ourselves comfortably in the relational space of the moment. Just think of all the folk expressions that refer to this: "Not having a leg to stand on," "Getting off on the right foot (or the wrong foot)," "Getting cold feet," "Being out of step," and so on.

Getting back to our apples . . . Now that we have found the right position, we can concretely fulfill our mission and achieve our goal: touching the apple, grabbing hold of it, and plucking it from the tree. We might then throw it away, or squash it, or bring it to our mouth, and so on.

Our upper limbs are the vector of action, expression, communication, strength, mastery, and control. Here we are in a relationship with action and realization (taking something in hand), whereas our lower limbs have a rapport with the relational.

The ills of our upper limbs can be a sign that we are experiencing tensions from our will to act upon the world—on someone or something; we are experiencing difficulties bringing our ideas and plans into reality.

Our trunk, our vertebral axis, and our spinal column are the place, where the coordination between the top and bottom takes place. Here, too, imagine that your trunk is fixed in place, and you can realize what role it plays in the discovery of space.

The vertebral axis and the spinal column are where the first impulse of movement originates, whether it comes from the head, the heart, the viscera, or elsewhere inside the body.

The hips and shoulders are the place from where the impulse leaves to be concretely manifested (impetus, enthusiasm).

The knees and elbows are the sites of flexibility and adaptation.

The hands and fingers, the feet and toes, all step in for the concrete realization of the act (at the end).*

Let's now take another look at the simple example of a pulled and aching muscle:

- It may have contracted into itself as the result of a direct assault such as from a punch, overwork, violent stretching, a surgical operation, and so on.
- Because muscles form chains, it could be suffering repercussions from other muscles (in various mechanical chains) as a result of reflex or analgesic interactions.
- It could be the influence of a visceral disruption through the "spider's web" of the fasciae.
- It is closely related to the skin (the reflex paths).
- Because it is part of an embryological construction (neuro-vertebral-organo-muscular), it is influenced by these different elements (an embryological and therefore energetic chain).
- Because it is a part of the body-mind continuum, it reflects the emotional and mental state of the individual. Any limitation placed on the full expression or realization of the action is inscribed through the body armor. Any internal tension is inscribed within the neuromuscular pattern.
- It could be the point targeted by the brain's "survival programming," connected to a certain feeling, experience, event, movement, or situation.
- Other options are also possible.

In Conclusion

Objectively speaking, in regard to the body, the organs, the cells, the atoms, the electrons, energy, emotions, thought, spirit, consciousness, where does one start and another end? "One train can hide another." We cannot place our trust in appearances! To quote Antoine de Saint'Exupéry: "The essential is invisible to the eyes, we only see clearly with the heart [and consciousness]."

---

*I can highly recommend two very intelligent books for anyone wishing to get a deeper understanding of these aspects. One is *Les Maladies, mémoires de l'évolution* [Diseases: Memories of Evolution] (Amyris Editions, 2004), by Dr. Robert Guinée. The other is *Dis-moi où tu as mal* [Tell Me Where It Hurts] (Albin Michel, 2003), by Michel Odoul.

PART TWO

Practical Work

9 • INTENTION AND APPROACH

To illustrate the state of mind that I suggest you adopt for working, I invite you to take a little walk discovering nature. To do this, you decide to take a little time to make your way to a natural nook, leaving your worries and cares behind and establishing contact with this countryside through your senses.

Naturally you will walk in a tranquil state of mind, sometimes slowing down or coming to a complete halt in order to hear one or more sounds with greater precision or to observe a natural detail more exactly. If you make the effort to examine things more closely, other details will appear to you.

You decide to explore this countryside using a footpath that cuts through it. Your awareness has been oriented by your intention to be open and receptive to observing life in all its facets and various levels using all of your senses. You are keenly aware of flavors, aromas, shapes, colors, and movements, of animal and plant life, and so on—all with an attitude of deep respect.

Your attraction to your surroundings is so profound that you remain unaware of the passing of time; the countless details that come to your attention only increase as your contact with the natural world grows deeper.

At the end of this little stroll, you feel recharged, your head has been freed from the normal buzz of thoughts and worries, and you feel a healthy sense of fatigue.

Now imagine this countryside as if you were marching briskly through it, your mind dwelling on your cares or on your plans for the future!

Slowing Down

When you establish conscious contact and allow it to naturally grow deeper, it leads you to move more slowly and sometimes even freeze to a halt. This is exactly what will happen with these massages.

The slow pace of this bodywork (or mind-body work) will be the expression of your intention, your attitude, and how deeply you are tuned in. At the same time it will encourage you to get settled and expand this contact more profoundly. You shall see that in the beginning it is really quite hard to work slowly—truly slowly.

Let's take a space that is several yards in length and filled with various shapes, colors, and aromas. With the speed of a rocket this space will quickly scroll before our eyes before we even have a chance to see or to feel it. In a race car, the countryside still rushes past fairly quickly, but we can rapidly catch a few elements of it. Now we are in a passenger car, peacefully moving down the road, and this small space begins to take shape. Next we pass through on a bicycle, and a lot of details appear, along with some odors.

Finally, we retrace our journey on foot. What a joy it is to be in contact with so many shapes, colors, smells, and movements—with all the life teeming in this small space. My advice to you is to make this journey on foot!

Pressure

Whether you press down firmly or lightly depends upon your intention. If you are seeking to focus on the skin, your touch will be gentle and light, like a caress. You may often be surprised not to feel anything, as if this space were anesthetized, nonliving, or uninhabited. You may react by spontaneously applying greater pressure, but now you will no longer feel the skin but the muscles instead, and this additional pressure runs the risk of quickly increasing their sensitivity.

As your skin awakens, you will have less and less need to press on it strongly, and the landscape it represents will become increasingly precise. If, mechanically speaking, you want to make contact with the muscular, fascial, or osseous space, then you will need to apply stronger pressure.

Different rates of pressure at varying speeds will permit you to explore the different levels of this landscape. But where are you going to go, and how will you get there?

Your Strategy

Let's take a rectangle to symbolize the zone you are going to explore. This space offers numerous possible ways to move. The essential thing is for you to spread your dragnet over the entirety of this space, the mesh of which can be ever smaller.

Let's look at one example: During your bodywork with a ball, you passed over a zone a little too quickly or too hard. This hurt and made you tense up to a certain extent. This zone is a kind of stumbling block. Now slowly go back over it—much more slowly. Deepen your awareness of this space that holds tension, as if you are an explorer who has spied a small piece of the countryside that greatly interests you, although it is hard to reach.

You will gently enter this countryside using its different elements for reference points: How painful is it? Where is it localized—is it in the muscle or in the bone? What kind of pain is it—does it hurt with a burning sensation, or is it more of a stabbing pain or like being caught in a vise? What words come to mind to best express it? Where is it most acute? These are but some of the questions that will arise.

What will permit you to start feeling at one with this zone and restoring it to harmony will be the attitude of gratitude, receptivity, and compassion you display toward this part of yourself. You are not imposing here: there is no adversary to fight, nor any intention to relax, to ease your tensions, stiffness, or pain. You are in a true listening space and are tuning in ever more deeply to what actually is. It is now that sensations, feelings, emotions, and images can really begin to surge up.

The self-touch therapy I am offering does not approach the body as if it were mere matter, a machine made up of different pieces, but addresses the life that inhabits the body directly (sensations, emotions, feelings, thoughts). It addresses the soul, the movement of life, that inner movement of growth that leans toward the realization of all your potential.

This discovery of the landscape can always be carried deeper. It is important to direct your intention toward the different aspects of the sensations that you are experiencing. This allows you not to evade but, to the contrary, to deepen this connection. This is the key for the success of this practice.

Pay attention to the automatism of your gestures. Do not repeat your movements at the same speed or with the same amplitude. This will put your "awareness" to sleep, and you will stop making any progress. The landscape changes with every passing second, and the sensations are different.

What detailed aspect of this landscape are you trying to uncover? I will give you a thread as a guide to help you find your way.

Exploring the Details in Depth

Open yourself to the sensation of mass (thickness, volume) and consistency (the hardness or softness of the tissues) of the skin, as this will help you feel the life in it. Then do the same for the fasciae (the membranes in which the muscles are wrapped), muscles, and bones. Each has its own distinctive consistency.

Open to other physical aspects, such as tension, relaxation, pain, pleasure, hot, cold, tingling, your heartbeat, and then go on into less physical realities, such as feeling charged, empty, or living, followed by feelings, thoughts, images, voice, color, emotions, and so on. Describing what you experience in a whisper in order to give greater precision to your sensations and feelings can be of great help.

Try to achieve a pace of infinite slowness for entering this landscape and, for example, transforming an irritatingly painful experience into an opening of this space, one in which you can simply let go and achieve physical and emotional integration. You can release an emotional charge through the liberation of the tissue without reliving the event that caused it or the emotion it generated.

Note: Your anatomical awareness is like a map you bring on your journey. It will guide you and allow you to explore places and details whose existence was unknown to you and where you would not otherwise be able to go. Do not confuse the image, the depiction on the map of this space, with the "felt consciousness" of this same space.

Implementation

Set aside some time just for you during which you will not be at the mercy of the telephone or other things that might solicit your attention; otherwise you will not be able to be completely available, which is crucial for establishing the receptivity that allows you to deepen your grasp of what you are feeling.

Put on some soft music as an accompaniment. It will mentally relax you and awaken your senses. Don't pick any music that will be too "soaring." In this bodywork approach we are primarily trying to establish a corporeal anchoring, and the one thing we are not trying to do is to escape our life space.

Find a small corner to work in. It should be between four and five feet wide, with nothing obstructing it, and open enough that you do not feel cramped.

Do not work directly on a tiled surface. If possible, work on a carpeted area, and do not hesitate to add additional layers of carpeting or a blanket to prevent any chill from the floor from reaching you.

It is not at all necessary to work directly on the skin. Just wear comfortable clothing that is warm and stretchy.

The Materials

These self-massages require the use of some fairly inexpensive objects that can easily be found in hardware stores and sporting goods shops. They are mainly tubes and balls of varying sizes and consistencies that can be easily adapted to meet the needs of the different parts of the body as well as the requirements of the intention.

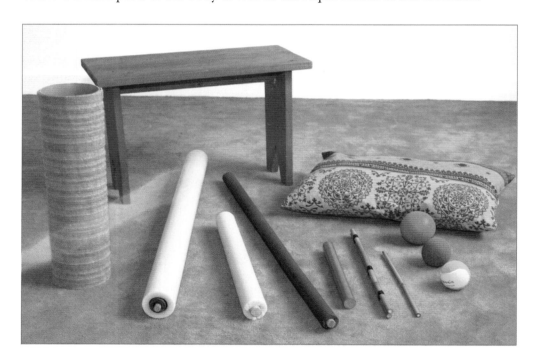

The Rollers
PVC Tubing
The tube should be around 130 mm (5 inches) in diameter and 70 cm (27 inches) long.

Cover the tube with a layer of thin carpeting or foam.

This material will provide firmness without being too hard on the body. It is essentially used to help you work certain parts of the lower limbs.

Foam Rollers

Foam rollers should be from 3 to 6 inches in diameter.

You can use pipe insulation as a foam roller. To give the insulation rigidity, slip a wooden pole inside. The size and rigidity of the foam rollers can be adapted for more delicate applications and for better working hard-to-reach places. For example, pipe insulation can be used without the pole in sensitive areas. Foam-covered PVC pipe also makes a good roller.

This tool will be used for different parts of the body.

The Balls

Balls allow you to provide more localized pressure and also to make contact with the deeper tissue layers.

There are two types of balls:

- Low-compression tennis balls made for children (balls made for adults are generally too hard)
- Foam balls, for a light workout over the skin and for deep draining of the abdominal area

You'll need balls of different diameters: a small ball that is about 6.5 cm (2½ inches), a medium ball that is 9.5 cm (close to 4 inches), and a large one that is 15 to 20 cm (around 6 to 8 inches).

The Rods

The rods can be made of bamboo or any dense, heavy wood, and they can be of different diameters depending on the zones that need to be worked. Chopsticks, thin curtain rods, and similar wooden wands are all appropriate.

With just these few basic tools, you can now massage yourself from head to toe without ever wearing yourself out!

10 • EXERCISES USING BALLS AND ROLLERS

This chapter will focus on exercises using the rollers and the balls (I will discuss the rods in a separate chapter). The exercises are accompanied by illustrations showing the relevant anatomical elements. I am providing you with detailed techniques for each part of the body:

- The head and neck
- The upper limbs
- The shoulders
- The chest
- The back and spinal column
- The belly
- The pelvis
- The lower limbs (thighs, lower legs, and feet)

Exercises for the Head and Neck

Skull and Neck

Seated

This exercise permits valuable work to be done on the entire back of the skull, the nape of the neck, and the neck itself. This position also makes it possible to

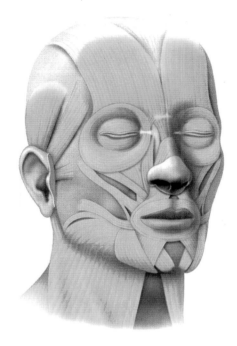

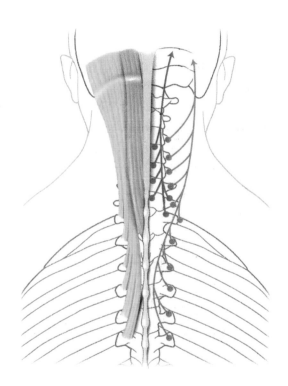

work on the region extending down the entire back to the lumbar region.

The pressure on the ball must be gentle.

Experiment with the foam balls to find which is easiest for you to use for this exercise. (For the back of the neck, the middle-sized ball often works best.)

1. Sit on a bench or stool with your buttocks and back pressed firmly against the wall. Place the ball directly behind your head.

2. Very gently and to the greatest extent possible, begin turning your head to the right and left, rolling the ball over onto the side of your head to facilitate the movement.

   The movement triggers a small bit of torsion in your torso on the side of the ball, as well as a slight tilting on the opposite side.

3. Place the middle-sized ball behind the nape of your neck, and once again turn your head slowly to the right and left.

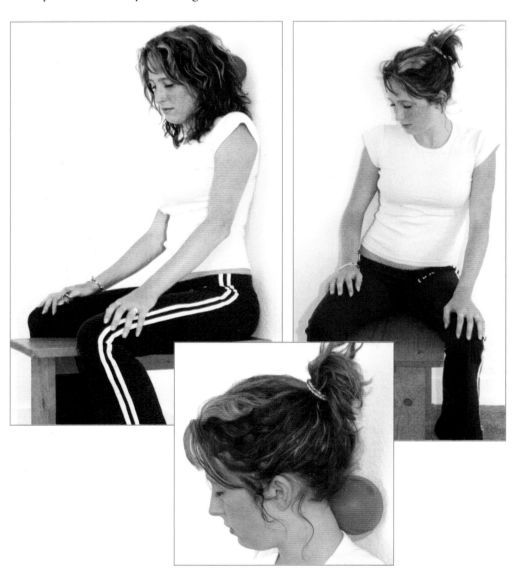

Standing

Performing this exercise in a standing position facilitates mobility and flexibility. With a little effort, it allows you to work the ball over your entire head and neck area.

Lying Down

Your mobility will be greatly reduced when performing this exercise while lying on your back, but this posture has the advantage of allowing greater relaxation and reducing the workload of the muscles. It allows you to work more specifically upon the base of the skull and the back of the neck.

1. Place your foam-covered roller under the back of your skull, as high as you can. It will give you the sensation that your neck is stretched.
2. Gently and calmly, begin turning your head from right to left (or vice versa) to discover the landscape of this area of your body.

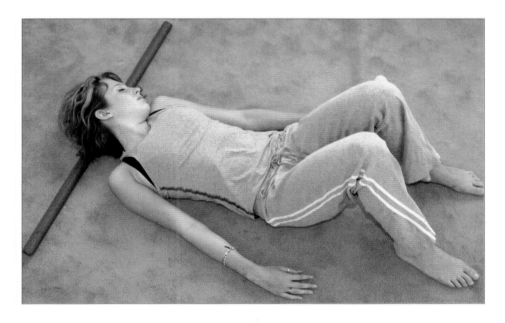

3. You can also roll the rod under your head from top to bottom. In this case, it can be placed a bit lower under your head.

4. Work the base of the skull and the back of the neck with the large foam ball.

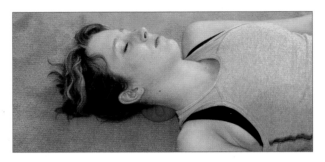

The Face

Seated

The small or medium-sized foam ball offer the most value here.

1. Sit down facing the wall with your knees open. Place the ball at the top of your forehead.
2. Turn your head from side to side to move the ball across your entire forehead.

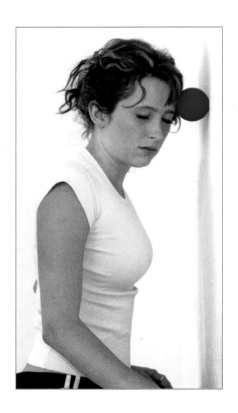

3. Bring the ball down to the level of your eyes, and again practice turning your head to move the ball across your face.

4. Move the ball down to the level of your nose, making sure to include your cheeks, followed by your jaws, mouth, chin, and wherever else your inspiration takes you.

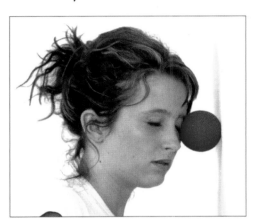 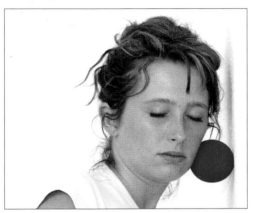

5. Move the bench or chair that you're sitting on a little back from the wall. Now, starting at the forehead, you will be able to massage the entire top of your head with the ball.

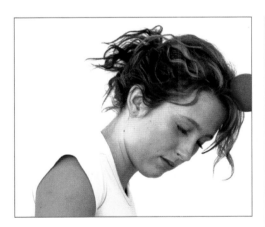 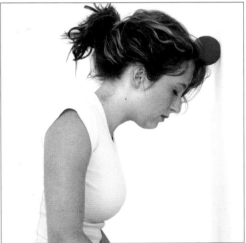

Exercises for the Upper Limbs

It is possible to work your upper limbs while either standing or lying down. Each of these positions will allow you to work more easily or with greater precision on different parts of your upper limbs. Balls or rollers can be used for this work. The balls are a bit trickier to handle but can provide significant results when used on the shoulder blades and the adjacent area.

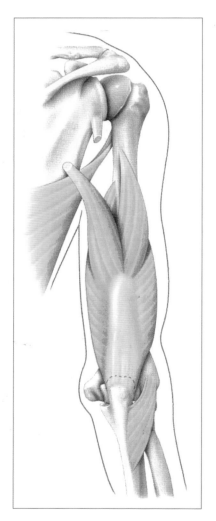 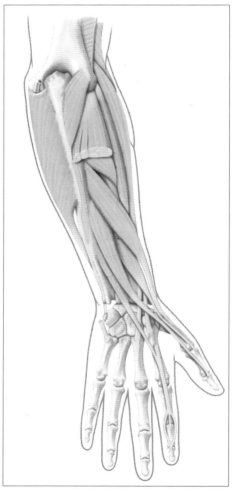

Standing

This position allows you to work on your entire arm.

1. Stand straight, facing the wall, with one of your forearms resting below your chest, over the thorax, and your other arm resting on top of the first arm in such a way that the whole area forms a rigid block. The palm of the upper hand should rest on top of the forearm of the lower arm.

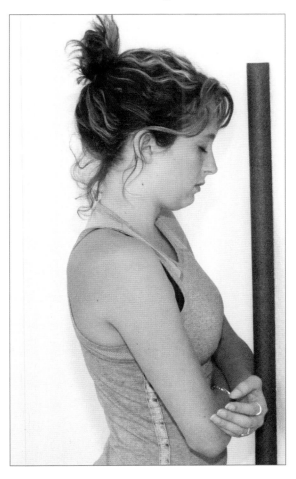 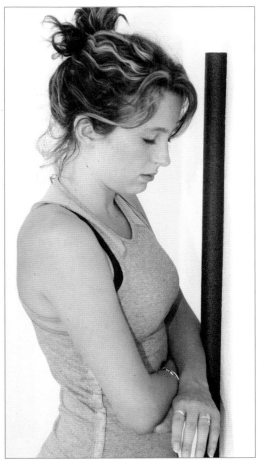

2. Leaning against the wall, twist your torso to create moving pressure on your arm. Start with the roller against the back of your upper hand, and let it traverse that entire area before shifting it onto the forearm.
3. To work on the outside of the forearm, turn your palm to face the ceiling.
4. To work the inside of the forearm, turn your palm to face the floor.

5. To work the upper arm with the roller, stand perpendicular to the wall, with your arms loosely crossed, so the arm being worked is not glued to your torso and your bodywork will not cause it to experience any tension.

6. Allow the roller to move up over the shoulder (the posterior deltoid) by turning your back to the wall. In this position you can then work your entire back.

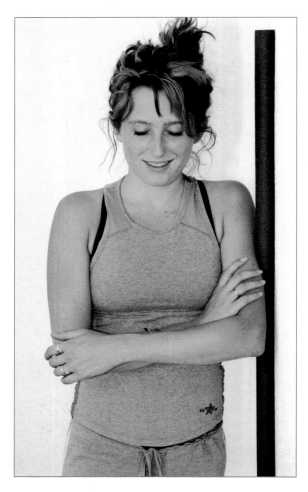 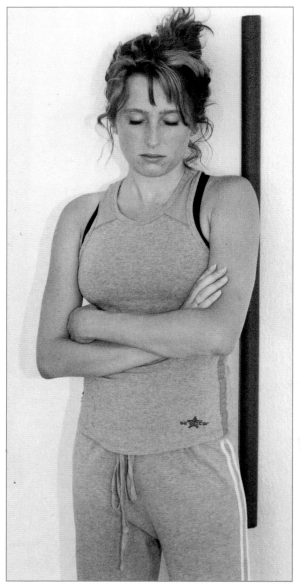

Lying Down

It is difficult to handle the ball when you are in this position. It is a much better idea to use the roller. Working while lying down is always of value, as it offers the greatest relaxation to your muscles.

1. Lie on your back with your upper arm resting on the ground and slanted away from your body. Place the roller so that it lies perpendicular to the back of the hand of the slanted arm, which is the arm you'll be working.
2. Roll your arm very slowly over the roller to explore its contact with this tool's surface.
3. In this fashion, bring the roller up from your hand, over your forearm, and up the rest of your arm until it reaches the shoulder (see page 88).

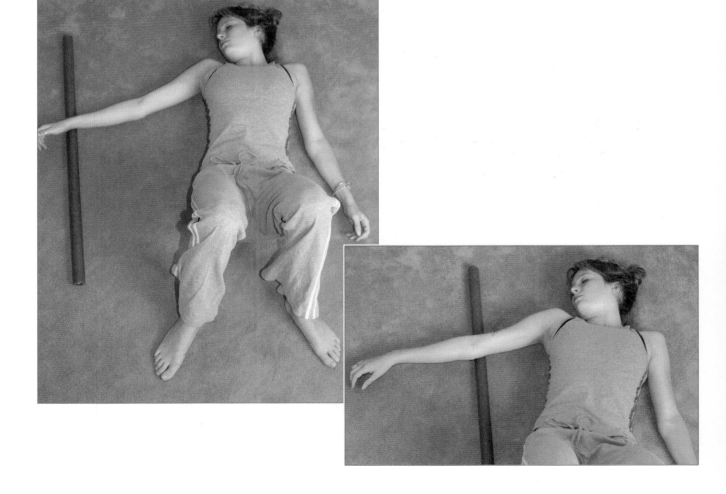

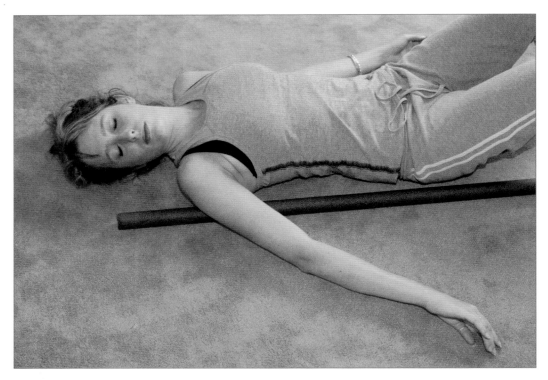

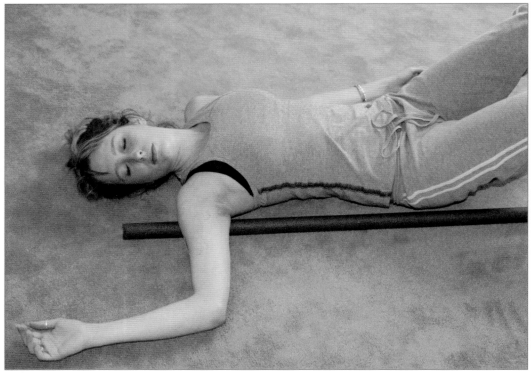

Exercises for the Shoulder

The shoulder is a zone that is technically difficult to massage and easy to hurt.

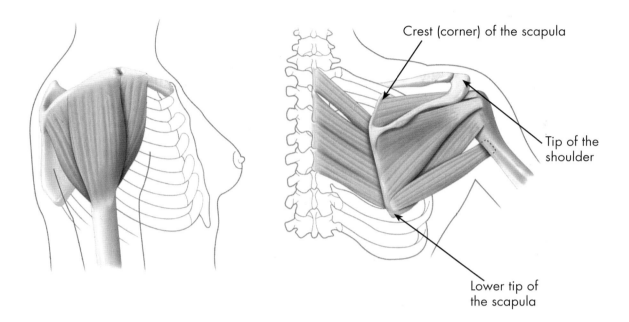

Crest (corner) of the scapula

Tip of the shoulder

Lower tip of the scapula

Seated or Standing

Use the medium-sized foam ball when massaging the upper part of the shoulder, above the shoulder blade, as it will stay in place and conform to your body's contour better than another tool.

The lower part of the shoulder, to the contrary, can be massaged with the different balls and the foam-covered roller.

1. Sit on a bench with your back against the wall and place the ball behind your spine at shoulder height (see page 90).
2. Perform a gentle twisting movement to move the ball from the center of your spine toward the tip of the shoulder.
3. Work one side first, then give yourself enough time to feel the difference the exercise has made before working the other side.

Caution: Don't press down so strongly on the ball that it becomes hard to roll. Because of both its size and consistency, the tennis ball is not suitable for use here.

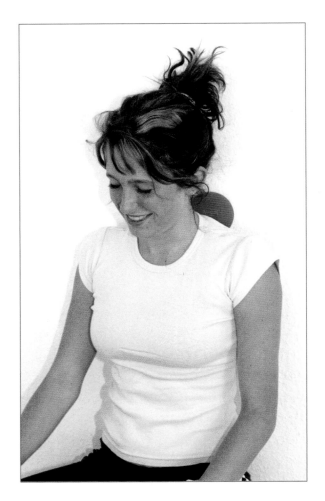

Lying Down

Place the foam ball or the foam roller (remove the rod from the center of the roller, if it has one) at different levels behind the shoulder, rolling it from the outside tip toward the scapular corner and to the lower tip. By "playing" with your arms and the ground, you will be able to modulate the pressure on the shoulder blade.

Exercises for the Chest

The chest is a zone that can be a tricky challenge to massage, emotionally speaking. From a more technical perspective, it involves very gentle and delicate work using a medium or large foam ball while standing up straight.

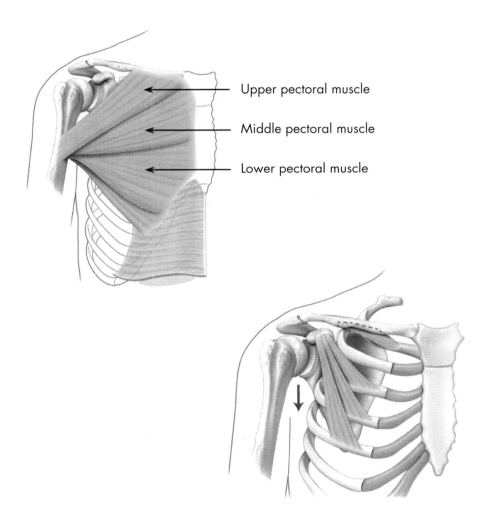

Upper pectoral muscle

Middle pectoral muscle

Lower pectoral muscle

Standing

1. Facing the wall, place the ball at the level of the sternum (see page 92).
2. Apply maximum pressure with your body to force the ball to roll very slowly, as if it were a caress, up toward the shoulder.

3. Use the ball to explore the upper part of your chest (beneath the collarbone), then the upper part of the breast, followed by the lower part of the breast.

For men the breast area corresponds to the upper, middle, and lower pectorals, which also exist in women but are partially concealed by their breasts.

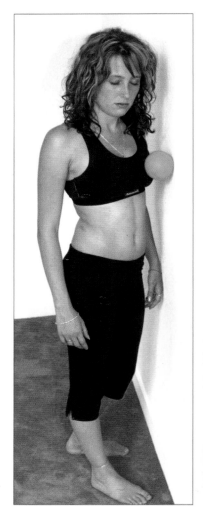
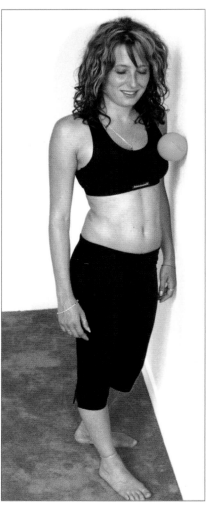
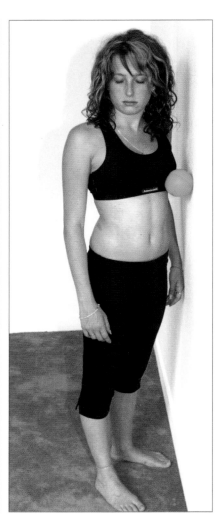

Exercises for the Whole Back

The back is a substantial zone for massage, containing many possible approaches that rely on balls and rollers, as each offers its specific advantage.

- The roller offers greater surface contact and therefore provides a more encompassing approach.
- Tennis balls are more limited in their range, but they allow you to massage a localized area with greater precision; they also allow direct contact with the deep tissue such as the bone, the periosteum, ligaments, and so forth.
- Foam balls can combine the more precise application of the tennis ball with a gentler pressure.

If your back aches or is sensitive, foam balls or rollers are preferable. There is too great a risk of applying too much pressure with the tennis ball and hurting yourself. In any event, it is well worth your while to experiment with the different tools, as the experience offered by each will expand your perception. See also the exercises for the head and neck (page 79).

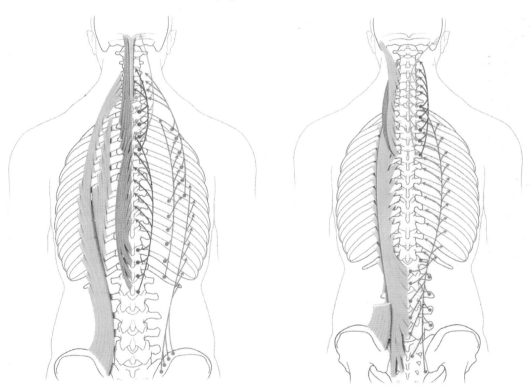

Standing

This position allows you a greater range of movement on either side of the back. The drawback is that your legs can become tired if you work on your back for too long.

With the Roller

I suggest that you first work one side from top to bottom, then pause to contemplate the difference the exercise has made before working on the other side.

1. Stand with your back to the wall, with the roller in a vertical position behind your head.
2. Keeping your back to the wall, move the roller down to the height of your shoulder blades. Shift your buttocks so that they are no longer pressed against the wall, leaving only the top of your back in contact with it.
3. Gently twisting your torso to move the roller, explore the zone between your spinal column and the tip of a shoulder.
4. Shift your base of support by standing a little straighter and bringing your buttocks back up against the wall. The pressure will now be strongest on the zone comprising the bottom tip of the shoulders and the lower ribs.
5. Make a twisting movement that will allow you to explore the entire surface of your back with the roller. You can shift the roller a little higher so that its lower end is at your waist and is not touching your buttocks, as shown in photo 1.

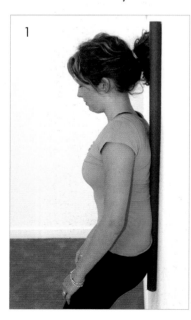
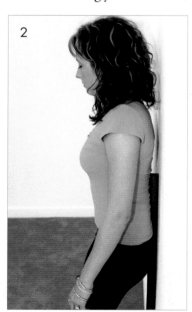
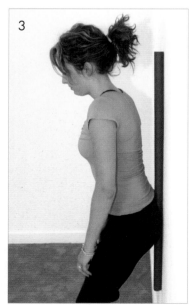

6. Shift the roller lower so that its top is now touching the top of the lumbar region (photo 2). The lumbar region can be a little difficult to work because you will need shift your body in such a way as to round it, so the roller can make contact with the entire lumbar surface.

7. End this exercise by working the roller over your buttocks (photo 3).

With the Ball

The protocol is exactly the same when using the ball.

Start with the ball behind your shoulder blade to work the sensitive muscles of this zone before moving down behind the shoulder, beneath the tip of the shoulder blade, and then down below the ribs until you reach the lumbar region.

Seated

Use a tennis or foam ball. By simply twisting your entire torso (you should feel a slight shift in support from one buttock to the other), you will be able to explore your entire back with the ball, from the top of your shoulders to the top of the lumbar region.

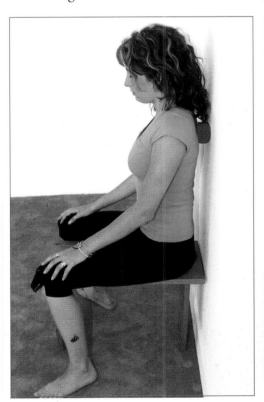
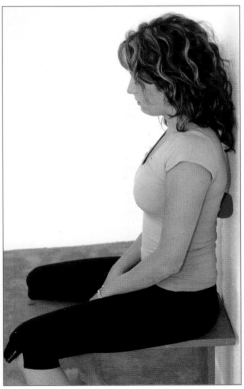

Exercises for the Spinal Column

Standing

You can provide a super massage over all the muscles that run along the spinal column from the base of the neck down to the sacrum. Work one side from top to bottom, then work the other side. The tennis ball is ideal here. You'll use the same technique to work all the levels of your back.

From the Base of the Neck to the Top of the Dorsal Muscles

1. Stand with your back against the wall, maintaining a gap between the wall and your buttocks. Place the ball between your spinal column and the inside edge of a shoulder blade.
2. Flexing your legs to move your body up and down, explore this region with the ball.
3. Move the ball laterally across this region by gently twisting your torso.

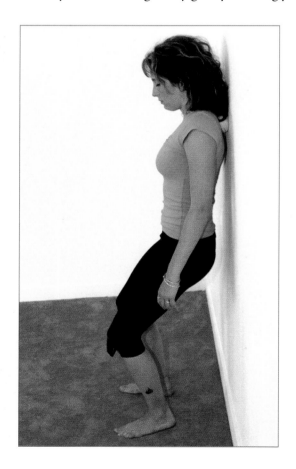

Between Your Shoulder Blades to the Base of the Dorsal Muscles

Using the ball, explore the region between the shoulder blades, from the top of the shoulder blades to the base of the dorsal muscles and from the lower tip of the shoulder blades to the lower ribs. You can work the ribs here as well.

The Lumbar Mass

You can work this voluminous and stimulating zone deeply when it is stretched out. Take advantage of this position to extend the work beyond this immediate zone onto the ribs.

The Sacrum and the Sacroiliac

Explore this area thoroughly both in length and in width. Put your intention on apprehending the bone here as well as capturing awareness of the muscle and ligament space.

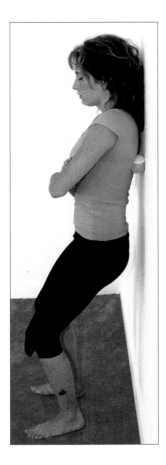
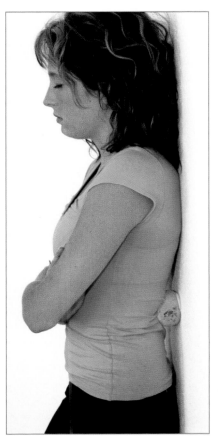
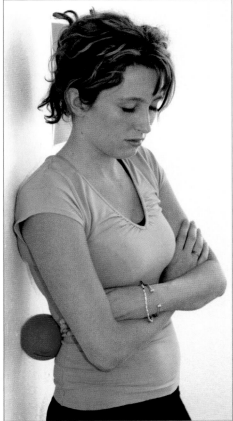

Note: To allow the ball to descend without using your hands, all you need to do is press your buttocks firmly against the wall and lean very slightly forward. If your back is quite sensitive or if you want to focus the contact on the skin and muscular envelope (the aponeuroses), use the foam ball.

Lying Down

Practicing the exercise in this position can be extremely rich in results and effective. Here you can use the roller or the tennis ball.

The Dorsal Zone

To work this region you will rely essentially on the roller. I advise you to remove any rod or tube that may have been inserted in the material, leaving just the foam.

1. Lie on your back with the roller perpendicular to your spinal column, at the level of the lower part of the shoulder blades. Extend your arms away from your body, so that they rest just above the roller. Bend your knees.

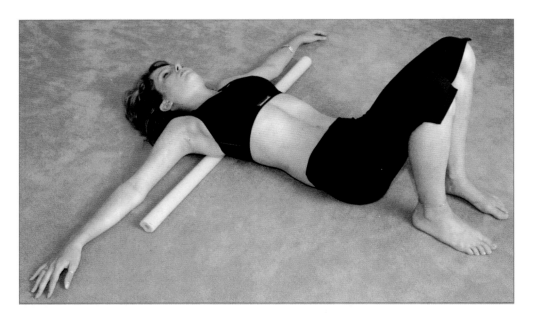

2. By bending and straightening your knees to a greater or lesser degree, you can move your body over the roller. By stages, cause the roller to descend your back until it reaches the base of the dorsal region.

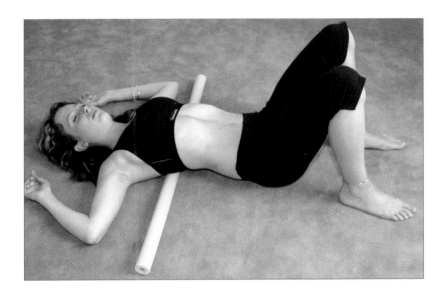

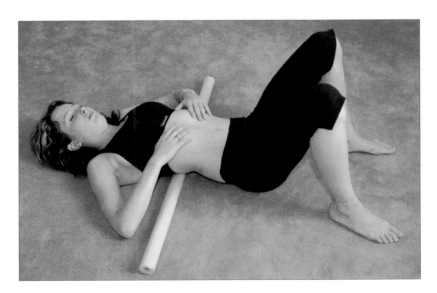

The Lumbar Zone

WITH THE BALL

The ball is a superb tool for working deeply on this area.

1. Lie on your back with your knees bent and your feet flat on the ground. Place the ball at the top of the lumbar region, several centimeters (a couple of inches) away from the spinal column.

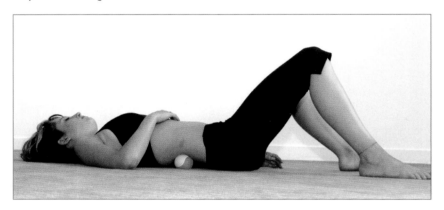

2. Bending your knees to a greater or lesser degree to move the ball down, and swaying them slightly from side to side to move it closer to and further from the spine, move the ball back and forth across the lumbar zone on one side of the spine, gradually descending. The pressure should not be irritating or painful; use the movement of your knees to modulate the pressure as necessary.

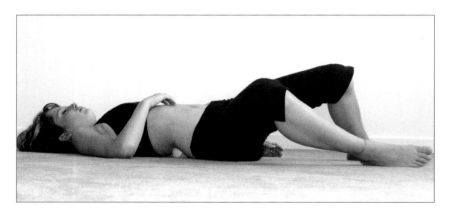

3. Before beginning this work on the other side of the spine, give yourself some time, with your legs stretched out, to feel the difference the exercise has made.

Note: I would like to remind you that it is very important to go as slowly as you possibly can in order to really "penetrate the details of the landscape" when moving through a painful space. This will allow you to unknot it, tame it, or simply be receptive toward it.

WITH THE ROLLER

The roller will allow you to work both sides of your back at once. Don't hesitate to remove the rod from the roller if your back is too sensitive to the support it provides.

Start with the roller at the top of the lumbar region, and move it down in several stages. Valuable results can be obtained by moving the roller continuously all the way to the base of the sacrum.

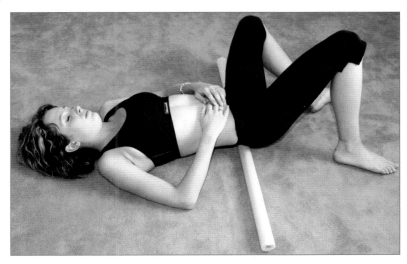

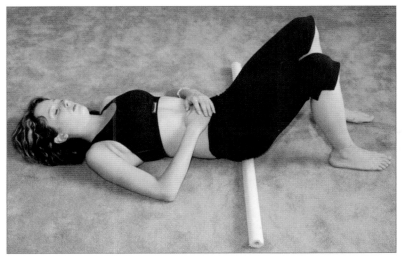

The Whole Spinal Column

WITH THE ROLLER

Here is a workout that is truly well worth the effort!

1. Lie on your back with the roller beneath you, parallel to your spinal column, running from the inner edge of the shoulder blade to the back of the hip joint. Your other side rests on the ground. Stretch out the leg on the same side as the roller; bend the leg on the other side, keeping that foot flat on the floor.

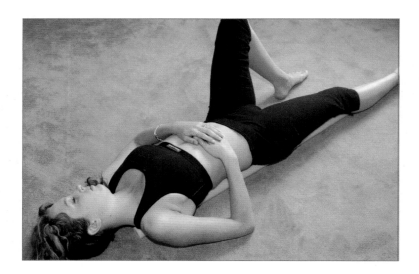

2. Lean your knees—particularly the flexed knee, on the side without the roller— from side to side to initiate a rotation of your pelvis and torso and apply the degree of pressure that you wish on the roller.

   Too much pressure, which is to say any degree of pressure that causes pain, will not allow you to tame and open this painful place. On the contrary, it will put you instead into a kind of conflicted state, a state of retreat and opposition to this part of your body.

3. Shift the roller a bit closer to your spine and perform this self-massage again. Then remove the roller and compare how your back feels on either side. You will be amazed at the difference!

4. Perform the same movements on the other side of your spine.

5. Place the roller directly under your spinal column, with the top beneath your head.

6. Explore this zone by making small oscillations with your body, slightly rocking at first and gradually making more ample movements, so that your back touches the ground on one side and then the other.

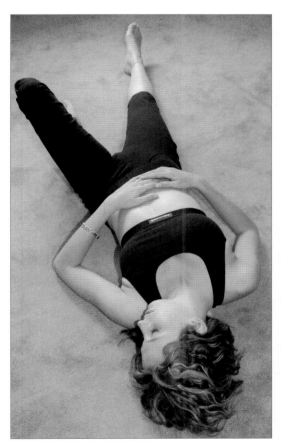 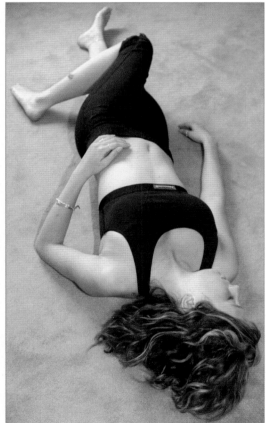

WITH THE BALL

Lie on your back with your knees bent and feet flat on the floor. Place the foam ball beneath your spinal column at the top of your back, and work it down your spine, stage by stage, until you reach the sacrum. At each stage, rock your body slightly back and forth to experiment with the sensations caused by the varying degrees of pressure.

Exercises for the Belly

What I am proposing for you to pursue here is making contact with your visceral organs through self-massage. In addition to its balancing effect and the expansion of bodily awareness to this region that it encourages, this work will cause a deep draining of the circulatory system as well as offering a gentle kneading effect on the intestines and other viscera.

This exercise is reliant upon ventral respiration (abdominal breathing), which creates a pressure from the inside moving outward, due to the push of the diaphragm during inhalation (this could be viewed as a piston that pushes back the visceral organs and inflates the belly), and a reverse effect when the diaphragm relaxes during exhalation. On the outside of the belly, the support of the ball creates inward-moving pressure, and resistance to outward movement.

You should use the foam ball when working your belly. The importance of the ball is twofold:

- It provides a counterresistance to the outward push made by the diaphragm.
- In certain spots (in correspondence with the organs), the support of the ball focuses the drive of the "piston" (the swelling of the belly, the sensation of a direct and clear pressure on the spot touching the ball) in a precise direction in relation to a specific organ.

This self-massage allows you to achieve a more precise and effective action on a specific organ. When you do this work, it's important that you understand a minimum of how the organ works—its shape, position, and role—so that you are able to picture it in your mind. You will find an anatomical illustration displaying the location of the abdominal organs on page 106.

1. Lie on your stomach, with the ball beneath you at the upper center of your belly, so that your body is tilted to one side. Bend the leg that is on the same side as the ball to modulate the pressure you feel.

    Imagine that your belly is divided into nine sections, as shown in the illustration on page 106. The ball should be in section 1.
2. Breathe into the ball, which is to say, allow your belly to swell outward when you inhale, as if you wanted the air to enter the ball and inflate it like a balloon.

What is important, and the chief difficulty with this exercise, is not to allow your entire belly to swell up but to orient and focus this inhalation on the spot in contact with the ball. This will clearly give you the sensation that you are directly pushing on this spot.

3. Take a half-dozen breaths with the ball in section 1. Then, taking a half-dozen breaths for each location, move through the sections, from 1 to 9, so that the ball moves from the left side to the right, beginning at the level of the stomach and ending with the navel.

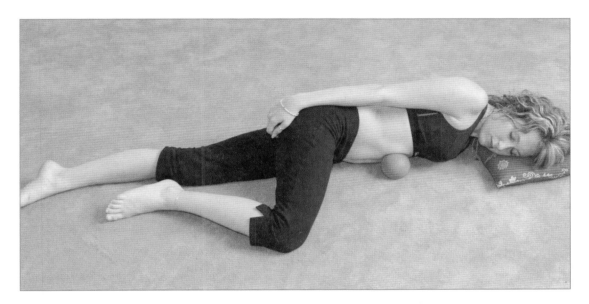

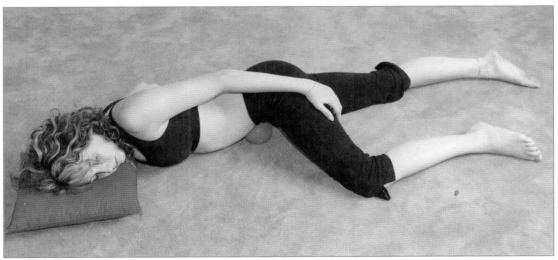

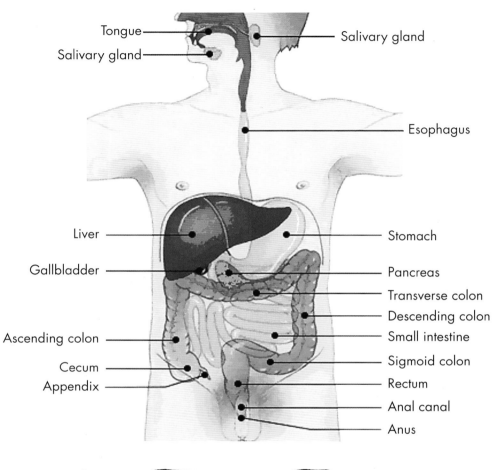

Tongue

Salivary gland

Salivary gland

Esophagus

Liver

Stomach

Gallbladder

Pancreas

Transverse colon

Descending colon

Ascending colon

Small intestine

Cecum

Sigmoid colon

Appendix

Rectum

Anal canal

Anus

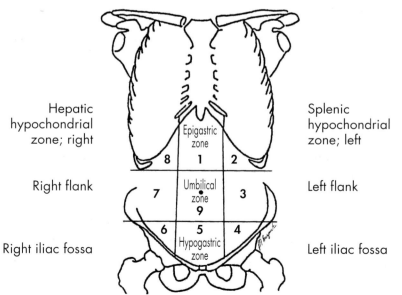

Hepatic
hypochondrial
zone; right

Splenic
hypochondrial
zone; left

Epigastric
zone

Right flank

Left flank

Umbilical
zone

Right iliac fossa

Left iliac fossa

Hypogastric
zone

8 1 2
7 9 3
6 5 4

The correspondence between the numbered zones and the organs	
1. Epigastric zone	The left lobe of the liver, the part of the stomach behind the liver
2. Left hypochondrial	Part of the stomach, the spleen, the tail of the pancreas, the left corner of the colon
3. Left flank	The descending colon, the intestinal loops
4 Left iliac fossa	The intestinal loops, the iliac colon, the left Fallopian tube, the left ovary
5. Hypogastric zone	The intestinal loops, the bladder
6. Right iliac fossa	The cecum, the ileocecal junction, the right Fallopian tube, the right ovary
7. Right flank	The ascending colon
8. Right hypochondrial	The right lobe of the liver, the gallbladder, the right corner of the colon
9. Umbilical zone	The transverse colon, the duodenum, the head of the pancreas, the intestinal loops

Exercises for the Pelvis

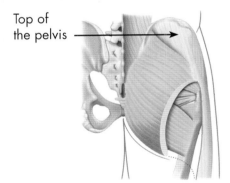

Top of the pelvis

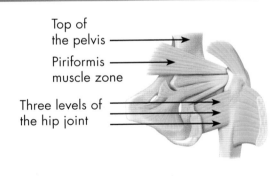

Top of the pelvis

Piriformis muscle zone

Three levels of the hip joint

This method of self-massage offers you a means of deeply working the area around the hip joints. A tennis ball works well here.

1. Lie on your back with your knees bent and your feet flat on the floor. Place the tennis ball beneath you, at the iliac crest at the top of the pelvis, about a hand's width away from the sacrum. Adjust the position as necessary so that it is not painful.

2. Rocking your knees to modulate the degree of pressure you are applying, initiate a sensorial exploration of this area, which will open the spaces that are the sites of blockages and pain.

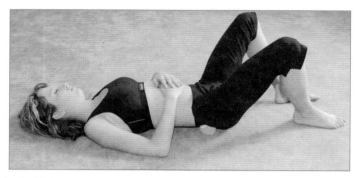

3. Move the ball down to the zone of the piriformis muscle, and work this area in the same way.

4. Bring the ball down behind the hip joint (coxofemoral joint), and work this area while descending over the three levels of this joint. Deepen your exploration so that you can feel the bone.

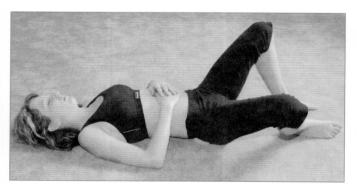 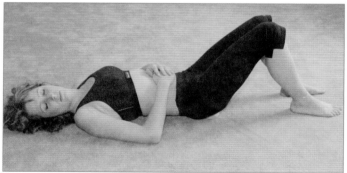

5. Move the ball down to the zone of the ischial spine, above the ischium (see the photos of the human skeleton, pages 132–33), and work this area in the same way.

Note: You can also perform this workout with your legs stretched out. Try it and feel the difference!

Perform this exercise on one side first, and allow yourself enough time to compare your two sides and to feel where the ground is supporting you, before working your other side. Do some stretches if you need to.

Exercises for the Lower Limbs: The Thighs

This area of your body offers a large variety of possibilities for working with all the different-sized balls and rollers. A large roller is a good choice for working on the back and inner surfaces of the thighs. For the front and outsides of the thighs, however, which are extremely sensitive areas, managing the pressure with a large roller is exhausting, and a small roller will work much better. It is often necessary to remove the central rod from the roller, if it has one.

I suggest you first work while lying down as this will involve all the surfaces of the thigh. Follow this with a workout while standing up to give more specific attention to the front and outsides of the thighs.

Lying Down
The Front of the Thighs

Here the small foam roller or tennis ball is called for. The latter is a trickier tool to manipulate here because of the larger amount of pressure it applies to a small surface but it allows you to work with more precision on a specific point or zone.

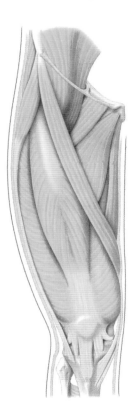

1. Lie on your stomach, with a small roller or tennis ball positioned beneath your thighs.

2. Explore the front of the thighs bit by bit, moving the roller or ball down by stages until it reaches just above the knees. You will be able to modulate the pressure you apply by the slight oscillation (rotation) of your torso.

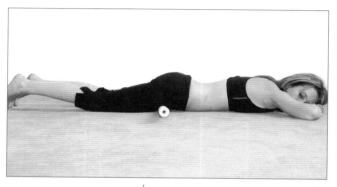 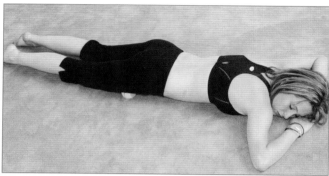

The Outside of the Thighs

The outer thighs have an extremely sensitive surface. Use a foam roller, with or without a central rod. The tennis ball can be quite valuable for working down the length of the thighbone. You can also use the foam balls if this zone is really sensitive, using the same principles.

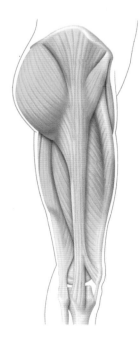

WITH THE ROLLER

1. Lie on your side in a comfortable position, with your head on a pillow or cushion. Position the roller beneath your bottom leg, perpendicular to the upper thigh, just beneath the trochanter (this is fairly high up on the front surface). Rest your upper leg on top of your lower leg.

2. Rock back and forth as gently as you possibly can by rolling your pelvis in order to shift the spot where the roller provides support. Do this several times.

3. Move the roller down a notch and start over. In this manner, explore the entire outer thigh region in five or six stages, down to the knee.

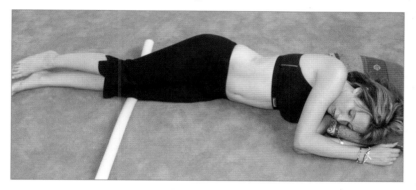

WITH THE BALL

Place the ball in such a way that it is not painful to perform this work. Note that when you roll the ball toward the front, it should press on the thighbone; if you place the ball too far back when you start, it will not be able to roll all the way to the bone.

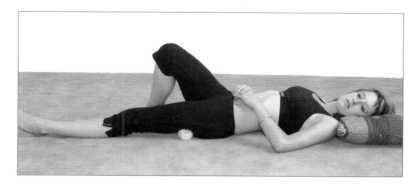

Note: This outer thigh zone, which does not have much muscle, is easy to hurt. Therefore, be careful to go very slowly here so as not to be caught unawares and cause yourself pain—that is not at all in the spirit of this approach.

The Inner Thighs

At the groin, the inner thigh is directly connected to the muscles surrounding the genitals. Any tension in these muscles will also express itself down the inside of the legs, so massage of the inner thighs will release blockages in the whole pelvic region.

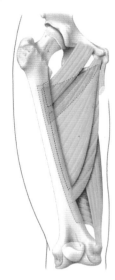

A large PVC or foam-covered roller is called for here.

1. Lie on your side in a comfortable position (don't hesitate to place a pillow on the ground for your head to rest on). Extend your top leg away from your body and bend your knee, so that the thigh is at a 90-degree angle to your torso, and the lower leg is at a 90-degree angle to your thigh. Place the roller beneath your thigh, perpendicular to it and just above the knee.
2. Rock very gently back and forth to gradually move the roller to the midthigh.
3. To explore the thigh up to the groin, begin with the roller at the midthigh level, and rock gently back and forth to slowly bring the roller up to the top of your thigh.

Note: This inner thigh zone is very stimulating, contrary to what some women think when they touch their inner thighs. The soft cushion they may feel is only the thickness of the skin and the fat that has accumulated there over the years. The muscles beneath that layer are often quite strained. A little bioharmonic "excursion" should help convince them!

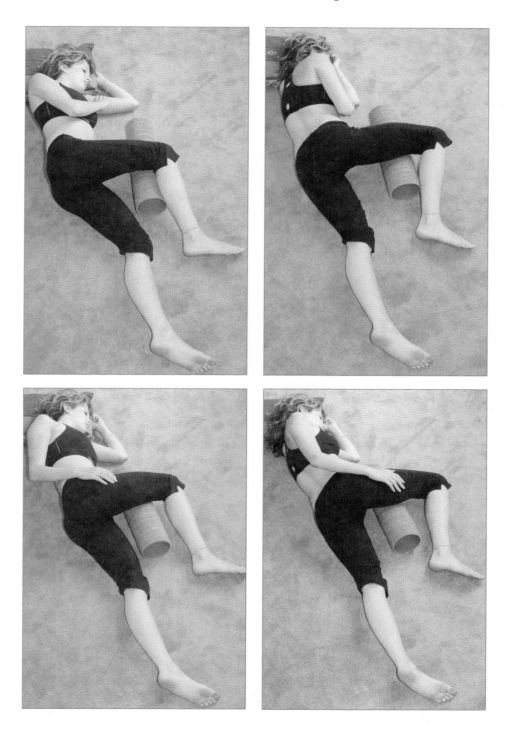

The Back of the Thighs

This zone is made up of large muscle masses, and working them can be quite stimulating. To work on the large muscles, use a large PVC or foam-covered roller. To work on the outer section, which is more bone than muscle, use the large ball.

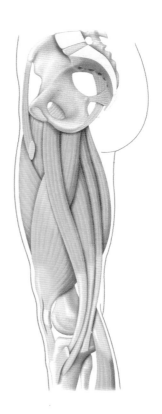

WITH THE ROLLER

You can use a large foam or PVC roller for this exercise.

1. Lie on your back; don't hesitate to place a pillow beneath your head if that helps you to be more comfortable. Bend the leg that you are not working, cross it over the leg you will be working in order to prevent it from tensing up. Place the roller beneath your upper thigh, perpendicular to your leg.

The weak pressure this tool provides allows you to easily contact the skin layer. If the pressure is too painful, use the foam roller and do not hesitate to remove the central rod.

2. By gently rocking back and forth, explore this region, moving the roller down in several stages until it reaches the hollow behind the knee.

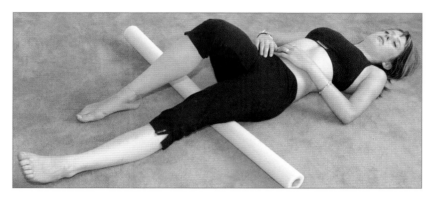

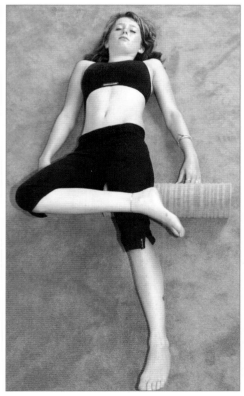
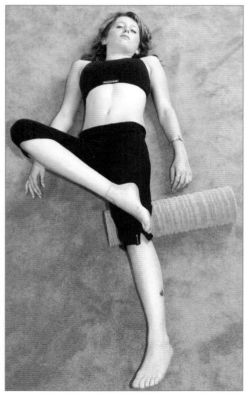

WITH THE BALL

1. Lie on your back, with the leg you are not working bent at the knee. Place the large foam ball just beneath the lower gluteal fold, behind the trochanter.
2. Rock your leg inward to modulate the pressure supplied by the ball. In stages, bring the ball down your leg until it reaches the knee.

Standing

The Thighbone

1. Stand with your side to the wall, with your foot directly against the wall. Position the ball between your upper thigh and the wall.
2. Move the ball laterally by twisting your torso. In this manner you can explore the thighbone at the front and side of the thigh, working from the top of the thigh to just above the knee.

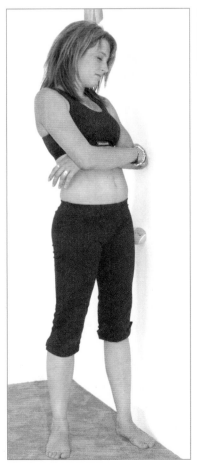
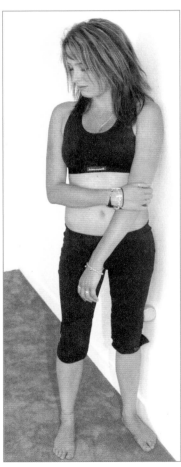

Exercises for the Lower Limbs: The Lower Legs

The lower legs are often quite "locked up," and blood and energy circulation through these zones can be quite poor and weak.

The Outer Calves

You can use either a ball or a foam roller here, each of these tools offering different qualities. Don't hesitate to vary the pleasures that discoveries of different sensations can bring! The protocol is the same regardless of which tool you choose.

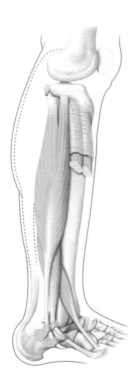

1. You have two choices of position for working the outer surface of the lower legs:

   - Curl up on the ground on your side, with your legs extended at a 90-degree angle to your torso and your knees bent, so that your lower legs are at a 90-degree angle to your thighs. Rest the upper leg on the lower one, or slightly behind it if that puts too much pressure on the leg you're working.
   - Lie on your back with your pelvis slightly rotated to the side you are going

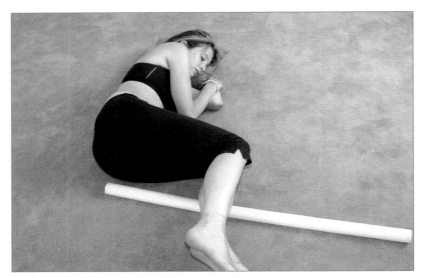

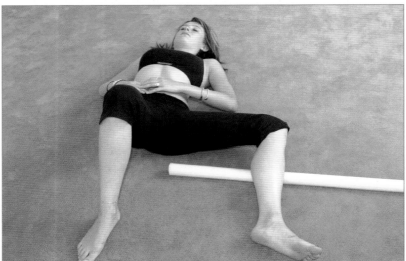

to work; hold it in this position by placing a cushion or pillow beneath your hip on the side you are not working. Drop the thigh of the leg you are working onto the ground, flexed at a 90-degree angle to your torso. Bend the leg you are not working at the knee, with your foot firmly planted on the ground or placed on the other leg as a means to increase the pressure provided by the support tool.

Place the roller at midcalf, perpendicular to the leg.

2. Use the roller to explore the upper half of your calf, from the midcalf to just below the knee.

3. Move the roller down to the level of your ankle, still perpendicular to your leg. Now explore the lower half of the calf, from the ankle to midcalf.

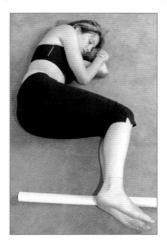

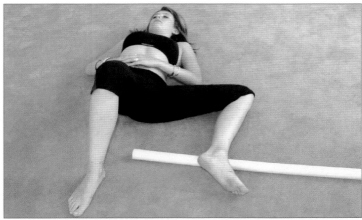

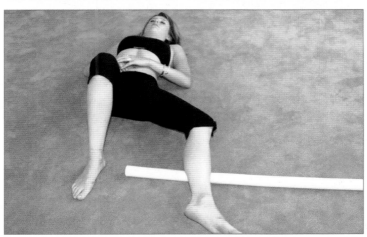

Note: The "landscape" of the outer calf has varied contours, and it is easy to inadvertently find painful areas.

The Inner Calves

You may use a large foam-covered or PVC roller, or even the different balls, for this exercise, depending on how sensitive this area is.

1. Curl up on the ground on your side, with the leg you are working extended at a 90-degree angle to your torso and your knee bent, so that your lower leg is at a 90-degree angle to your thigh. Let your bottom leg stretch out straight, resting on the ground.

   To explore the upper part of this surface area, place the roller or ball beneath your lower leg, at the midcalf level.

2. Use the roller or ball to explore the upper part of the inner calf, from the midcalf to just below the knee.

3. Place the roller or ball at ankle level, and use it to explore the lower half of the inner calf, from the ankle to midcalf.

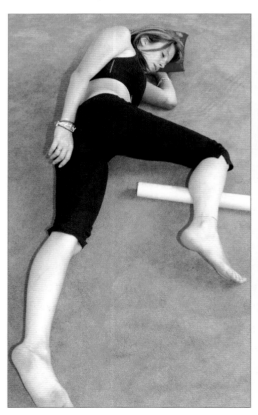
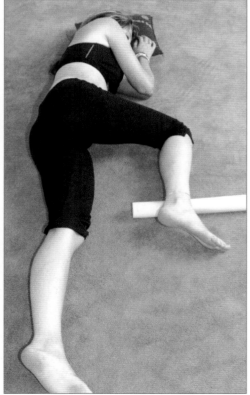

Note: As the inner calf is often an extremely sensitive zone, the midsize foam ball often proves to be the best choice for working here.

The Front of the Lower Legs

There is not a wide range of possibilities for working on the shin area. Your best option is to choose the large roller, as here the ball would provide a difficult technical challenge.

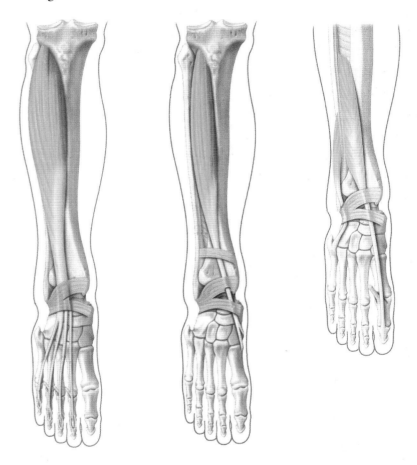

1. Curl up on the ground on your side, making sure the arm beneath your torso is in a comfortable position. Don't hesitate to put a cushion or pillow under your head if that helps you to be more comfortable. Your legs should be extended at a 90-degree angle to your torso, and your knees should be bent, so that your lower legs are at a 90-degree angle to your thighs. Let your top leg rest on the bottom

leg, bending your knee slightly so that the back of your top foot touches the heel of the bottom foot.

From this position, you'll be working your bottom leg. Position the roller beneath the upper part of that shin, perpendicular to it.

2. Gently rock your torso and pelvis back and forth to explore the upper shin zone with the roller.

3. Bring the roller down in several stages, from the upper shin to the ankle. At each level, experiment with the rotation of your legs.

Note: The shin surface is also extremely sensitive.

The Back of the Lower Legs (Calves)

You should use a large foam roller here (the PVC roller is too hard), and I advise you to remove its center rod if it has one. A large foam ball could be used here as well.

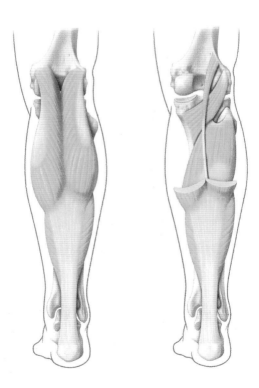

When you begin, the pressure on your leg at the top of your calf could be intense, but it should lessen as the roller descends toward your ankle. This exercise is quite useful for working on the Achilles' tendon and heel and can produce some very worthwhile results.

1. Lie on your back, with a pillow beneath your head if necessary to make yourself comfortable. Position the roller beneath and perpendicular to the leg you intend to work, just below the knee. Bend the leg you will not be working, setting that foot flat on the floor or crossing that leg over the leg you will be working.
2. By rocking your pelvis back and forth, explore this region of the calf supported by the roller.
3. Bring the roller down your leg in stages, stopping to explore the area behind the upper calf, the rounded area of the calf, the base of the Achilles' tendon, and finally, the heel (also see page 124).

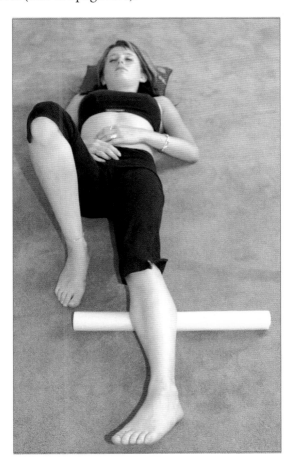

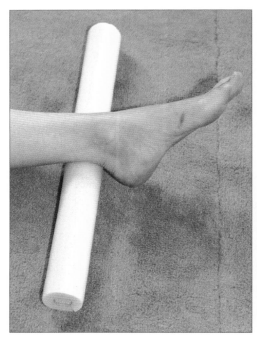 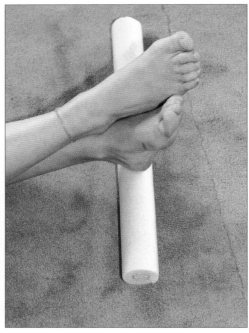

Note: The calf can be extremely sensitive in certain places. Don't be too aggressive, and explore this region very gradually, as this landscape is full of pitfalls!

Exercises for the Lower Limbs: The Feet

Your feet are an important area with which to make contact. You can work on them while seated, standing, or lying down, and you can use either the ball or the roller. Here, as is the case with all the other exercises, the purpose is not to provide a reflexology treatment (in other words, to massage a specific point in order to cause an effect on an organ or body function), but to simply "inhabit" this zone (and to trigger all the synchronizing processes that will flow out of the extension of your awareness into this area). This contact will inspire a mechanical and even a reflexology effect, although that was not the specific intention.

There are two ways you may proceed:

- Roll the ball or roller beneath your foot.
- Move your foot over the ball or roller, which has been fixed so it will not move.

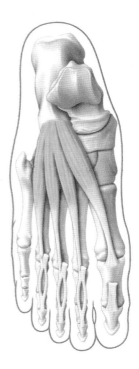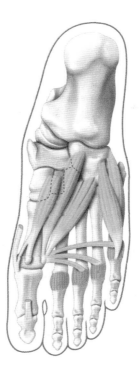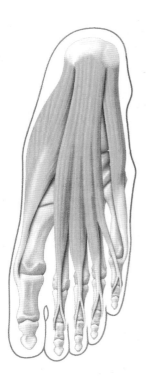

If you work your feet one after the other, it is always a good idea, before doing the second foot, to stand up and compare the sensations and sense of support on each side of your body.

Seated

Here, you can work on both feet at the same time or one foot at a time. The protocol to follow is the same with either the ball or the roller. You could also use a wooden rod instead of a roller. But be careful not to be too aggressive and hurt yourself!

1. Sitting on a stool, bench, or chair, place the ball or roller beneath your foot; if you're using the roller, it should be perpendicular to your foot. This position ensures that the pressure is quite light, which will permit you to connect with and extend awareness into the skin or surface muscles especially.

   If you are working just one side, you can increase the pressure applied by the support tool by crossing the leg you are *not* working over the leg you *are* working, high enough that the support tool is the only thing supporting the foot you are working.

2. Use your foot to roll the roller or ball around very slowly as you explore this zone.

- Keep your knees straight for the roller or ball to make contact with the middle part of your foot.
- Open your knees outward to explore the outer part of your foot, including the outer edge.
- Pull your knees in to explore the inner part of your foot, including the inside edge.

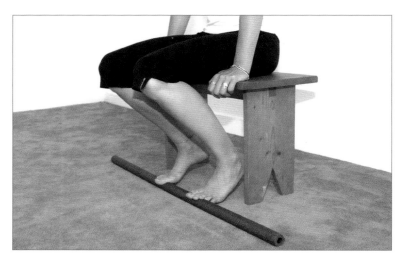

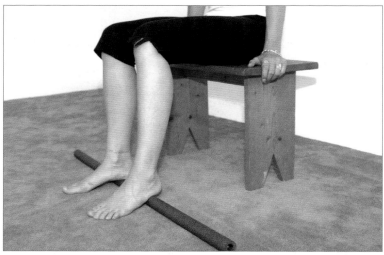

You can perform this exercise as a regular exploration, or you can use it to refine your sense of what you've already discovered by stopping to focus on one point, varying the degree of pressure you apply to it.

Once you have stopped on one specific point, simply lean forward, with your elbows braced on both knees. If you are working on just one side, gradually shift the support of your torso until it is entirely over that side. If your seat allows it, you can make it sway toward the front to modulate the pressure even more.

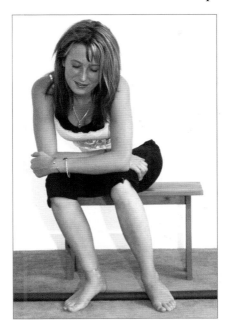

Note: Try to generate small, gentle sensations in your feet that will allow you to deepen and refine your awareness.

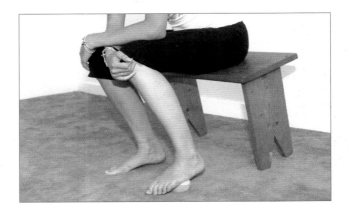

Standing

With the Roller

Standing up allows you to provide strong pressure to your feet, so be careful! You can remove the central rod from the roller if your feet are sensitive. You'll work on one foot at a time here. After you've worked on one foot, before moving on to the second, take a moment to compare how your feet and legs feel, and the support your body feels from either side.

1. Stand with your legs spread and the roller beneath the heel of one foot, perpendicular to it.
2. Gently rock back and forth several times to modulate the pressure on the foot. Find the slowest pace you can maintain.

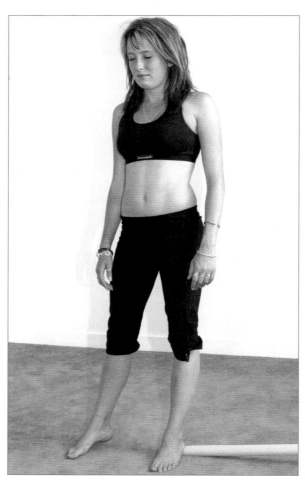

3. Move the roller slightly forward, and rock back and forth to explore this spot. Continue in this manner until the roller has reached the base of your toes.
   You can create different series of movements with the rod by following various lines of support: heel to third toe, heel to big toe, heel to third toe.

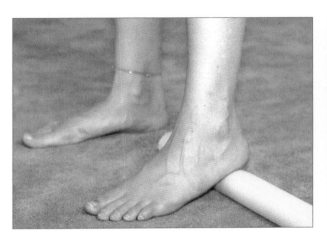 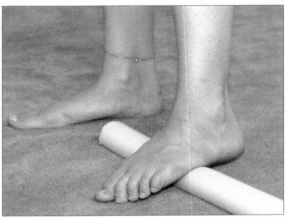

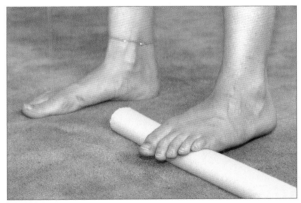

With the Ball

Follow the same protocol used with the roller.

Note: It is simply the oscillation and gradual transfer of the weight of your body that creates the variation of pressure on your foot. There is no need to intentionally push down, or to contract your thigh or leg to increase the pressure supplied by the roller or ball. Keep your knee straight, as this will allow for the suitable amount of weight to be transferred onto the ball.

The Arch of the Foot

1. Lie on your back. Put the foot you intend to work flat on the ground, with the knee bent; let your other leg lie flat on the ground. Place the roller beneath the arch of your foot, at the heel, and extending under the calf of your straight leg.

2. Explore the arch of your foot simply by gently rocking your knee back and forth. Bring your foot down over the roller in stages until it reaches the base of your toes.

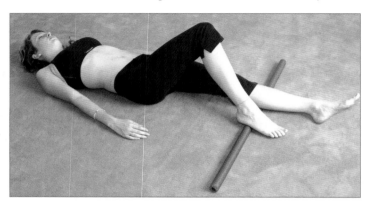

The Outer Edge of the Foot

1. Lie on your back, with a pillow under your head for comfort, if necessary. Twist your pelvis to the side, and slide a cushion under the raised hip to maintain this position. Let your bottom leg rest on the ground, with the knee bent and your foot on top of the roller, which should be in a perpendicular position. Your top leg can rest on top of the bottom leg, or you can raise the knee on that leg, resting its heel on the heel of your bottom leg, in order to increase the pressure on the outside edge of your bottom foot.

2. Slide your leg and rock your foot to explore the pressure of the roller on this area.

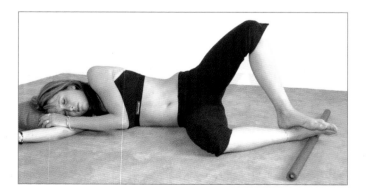

11 • EXERCISES USING RODS

Rods, in the context in which we are using them, can be seen as extensions of the hands that make it easier to work without tiring and to be more receptive by virtue of the judicious use of your arms and the rest of your body.

Working with rods adds immeasurably to the means we have at our disposal to discover the landscape that is our body. They particularly make it possible to explore the skin more delicately by scratching, sliding, and rubbing. They can also be used to work the bones and the (anatomically) deep places using vibratory techniques.

Whether you are using balls, rollers, or rods, it is very important, in order to get the utmost benefit from this body-mind work, to find the most comfortable position possible so you do not have to make any effort that would work against the state of consciousness you are seeking to attain. This helps you move the most active part of your mind into the background and become totally focused on becoming receptive to yourself through your sensations.

The Techniques

Vibrations

Sometimes you need to work on a spot where the bone does not lie too deeply beneath the skin. This rod technique is a splendid tool for this kind of bodywork. It makes use of the properties of vibrations, which spread out from the point of impact. When applied to a bone, vibrations not only spread through that bone and all the bones connected to it but also fan out into the surrounding tissue.

Your intention when beginning this exercise is to send out a vibration, like a tiny breath that crosses through a space, awakening it and inducing it to feel. The impact must be strong enough to reach the bone and echo. The force used here will therefore depend on how thick the skin is at the place on which you are working. If it is too thick, the impact necessary to reach the bone will be too strong and therefore counterproductive.

Do not create too many vibrations in succession, as this creates the risk of overloading the space with vibrations instead of lightening and relieving it, and you will therefore not achieve the harmonizing effect you are looking for.

Just give yourself a little light, firm "flick" with the tip of the rod, wait several seconds, which is how much time you need to feel the vibrational effect spread, and do it again at the same place or at a spot a little farther away.

This impact will spread in both distance and depth, even if it cannot be felt. You must direct your attention to focusing on the part of your body you are working, and let the sensation arrive. If you do not really know how you are put together anatomically, you will not be able to truly awaken the consciousness of that zone. Here is where a little anatomical knowledge will help you in performing your self-massages, like the explorer who has a detailed map of the countryside that lets him orient himself and reach a specific point.

As a reference in this regard, here are several photos of our human skeleton.

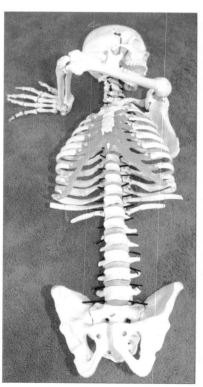 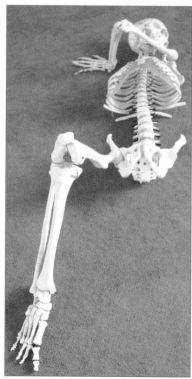

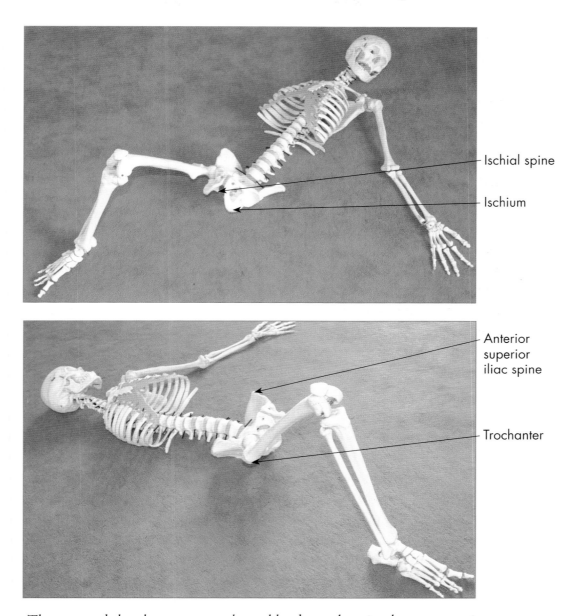

Ischial spine

Ischium

Anterior superior iliac spine

Trochanter

The map and the photos are not the real landscape but simple representations. Nevertheless, they can be of real assistance. But do not confuse the image—the depiction you have in your head—with the sensations you are feeling.

Note: In this book I am suggesting ways that you can awaken your bones through vibrational techniques, but you can also use these same techniques to cause the skin or muscles to vibrate, using more or less the same positions.

Scratching, Sliding, Rubbing

These movements are made very lightly. The intention here is reawaken your awareness of your bodily sensation, to help you feel the skin both on its surface and in the depths of its thickness. These massages are generally performed with the very tip of the stick or rod.

Exercises Using Vibrations from Rods

The Skull and Face

This area provides a particularly interesting area for this kind of massage. There are many possibilities for "excursions" here. What I can provide you with is the major route.

1. Stretch out comfortably on your back. Hold the rod in one hand near your face, with the elbow of that arm on the ground; you can sandwich a cushion between your upper arm and forearm to cut down on the muscular exertion that would otherwise be required. Turn your head slightly to the side of the rod.

    I suggest that you hold the rod in the middle, as seen in the photos below and on page 135. All the movement is propelled by a slight flick of the wrist. Your fingers should not grip the rod tightly; instead, leave a little play in your grip to facilitate the little rebound the rod will make after the moment of impact. The gentler and lighter the gesture—just firm enough to let it resonate in the bone—the greater your chance of having a vibration that "opens" you and creates a harmonizing, synchronizing effect.

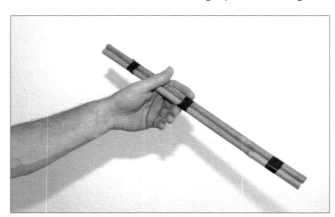
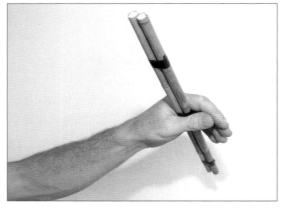

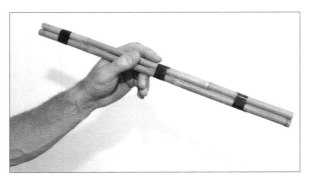
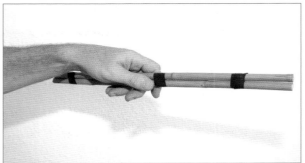

2. Work the side of the face on the same side as the hand holding the rod. Start between your eyes and radiate out over the forehead and the top of your head, the bridge of your nose, your cheek, the chin, and around the jaw.

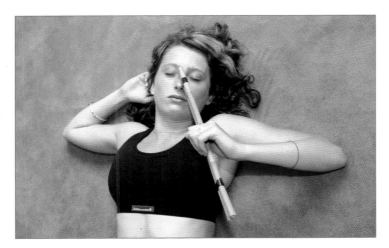

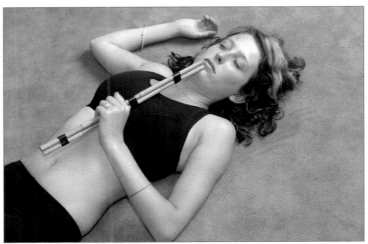

3. To work the side of the face that is opposite the hand holding the rod, ideally you would hold the rod in your other hand, but when it comes to dexterity we all have a "right" and a "left" hand, so if necessary you can instead simply turn your head sharply.

Note: For vibrations in particular, do not remain focused in your intention and awareness on the spot of impact. Accept feeling the resonance of the impact as it travels in distance and depth.

The Thorax

This zone is very emotionally charged. Do not invade it with strong vibrations.

1. Lie on your back with your knees bent and the elbow of the arm that holds the rod resting on the ground.
2. Make tiny "flicks" of the rod on your sternum, going up from the bottom to the top, if you can. Men tend to have less difficulty than women finding appropriate impact zones.

   Feel the bone in both its thickness and its length. Make a tiny flick on the upper ridge of the sternum. The vibration caused here will naturally radiate into the ribs, toward the dorsal vertebrae. You will therefore be able to "capture" these different levels.

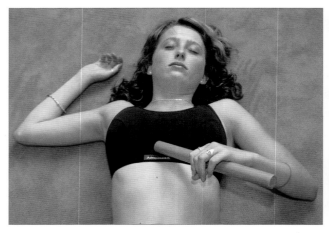 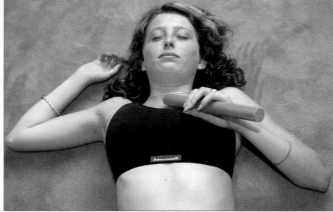

The Clavicle

Once you have reached the top of the sternum, continue your sensory exploration with the clavicle, from its inner end all the way to its outermost border, which ends just before the tip of the shoulder. If possible, hold the rod with the hand opposite to the area you are exploring so that this zone will be as undisturbed and peaceful as possible.

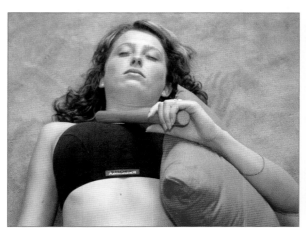 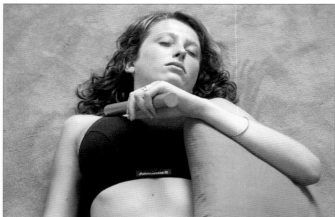

The Tip of the Shoulder and Shoulder Blade

Lying on your side in order to disengage your shoulder blade, and with your elbow braced on the ground in order not to tire your arm, start your exploration at the tip of your shoulder. From here, move toward the inner edge of the shoulder blade with the intention of apprehending the space occupied by this bone.

You can continue working on this same side all the way down to your hand, or you can work on the opposing clavicle and shoulder blade.

The Upper Arm

It is hard to make effective impacts along the length of the humerus bone, as very little of it is close to the skin surface. Instead, concentrate your efforts at the top and bottom of the bone.

1. Flick the tip of the shoulder with the rod, directing the impact down the length of the humerus bone, with the intention of feeling the reality of this bone mass.

2. Grasp your opposite shoulder with your hand, resting your elbow on your chest. Flick the tip of the elbow, directing the impact into the axis of the bone.

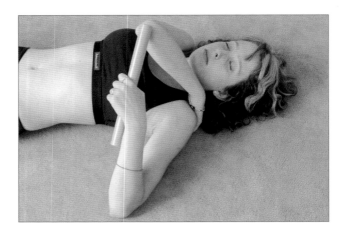

The Forearm

1. Raise your arm up next to your head, with the elbow bent and pointing up. Flick the tip of the elbow, directing the impact toward the axis of your forearm (the radius and ulna).

2. Resume the position you used for working on the upper arm, and work your way down the forearm to the hand.

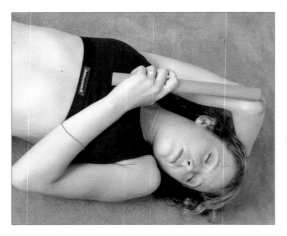 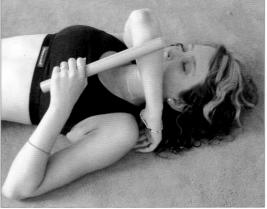

The Hand

This zone offers many bone areas right beneath the skin, which makes it possible to explore all the spaces of the hand in greater detail than in many other parts of the body.

When exploring your fingers, you could use more delicate and slender tools, such as wands.

1. Flick the ends of your extended fingers and/or your nails, directing the impact down the finger axis. This impact should be small but sharp; do not strike too strongly.

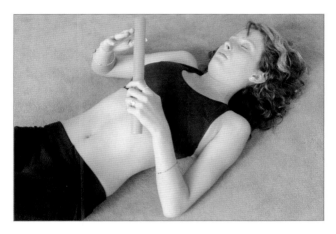

2. Flex the joint between the first and second phalanges of your fingers. Flick this joint, again directing the impact down the axis of the finger.
3. Flex the joint between the metacarpals and the first phalanges. Flick this joint, directing the impact into the metacarpus.

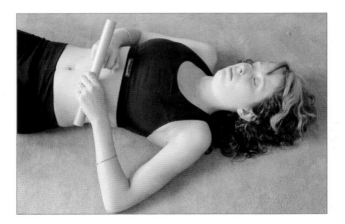

These vibrations will radiate outward to some distance. It is interesting to finish this exploration of your arms by seeking to apprehend, via the bone, this sensation globally all the way into the shoulder blade, the collarbone, and even further.

The Spinal Column

Making an impact directly upon the vertebrae would require too much acrobatic movement and exertion, which works against achieving the letting-go state necessary to realize the benefits of this massage. On the other hand, it is possible to work on this area from a distance. To work on the dorsal vertebrae, the point of impact should be on the sternum. The impact that will affect the pelvis needs to be made on the knees and the anterior superior iliac spine (ASIS) of the pelvis.

The Pelvis

There are two possible impact zones:

- The anterior superior iliac spine of the pelvis
- The trochanter, which is often harder to access because of its "wrapping" (see the photos of the skeleton on pages 132–33).

1. Stretch out on your back with your knees bent in order to relax the tensions at play in this area.
2. Explore this pelvic area with vibrational flicks. The direction in which the vibrations travel will depending on the direction of the impact. Regardless, the vibrations will spread throughout the pelvic area, even if you do not feel it.

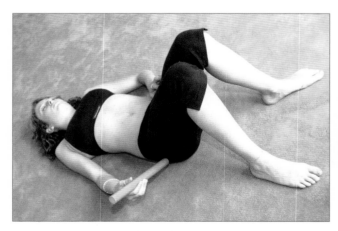 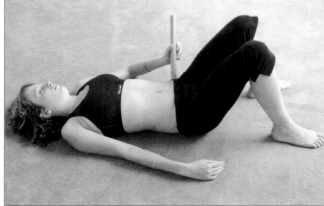

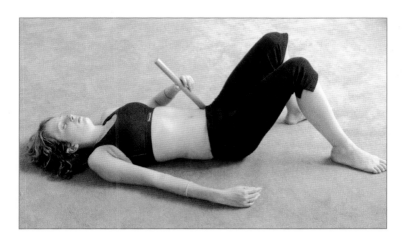

The Lower Limbs

This is a good zone for working with vibrations, which are especially beneficial for circulation. I suggest that you start your massage at your feet and work up toward your knees. You may work seated or lying down; the prone position is always worthwhile, as it encourages relaxation and helps you to tune in.

Lying Down 1

1. Stretch out in a comfortable position, with one leg bent and the other crossed over it, with the knee open.
2. Work the raised foot with vibrational flicks from the inner edge of the big toe and along the foot up to the malleolus (the small, rounded prominence on the side of the ankle). Work up your lower leg, following the crest of the tibia, until you reach your knee.

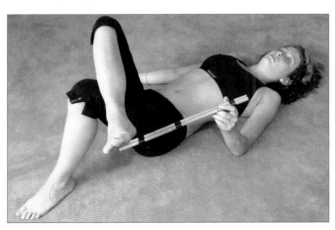
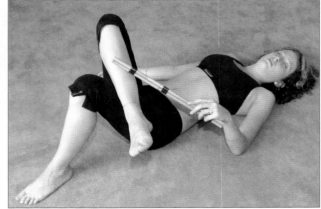

3. Working on the knee with vibrations is quite worthwhile, as it allows you to direct the vibrations down the tibia toward the feet (the impact should be above the kneecap, along the axis of the tibia) or down the femur toward the pelvis and spine (the impact should be below the kneecap, along the axis of the femur). Practice working the knee in both directions.

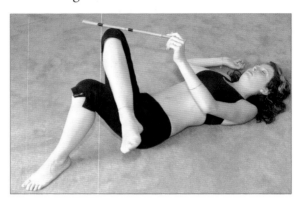

Lying Down 2

Lie on your back with your knees bent and your feet flat on the ground. Work up the lower leg from the ankle to the knee. Experiment with working both the back of the leg and the front of the leg. This position allows you to work the impact more upon the knee.

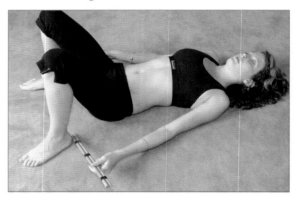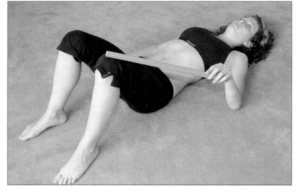

Seated

This position allows you to work the entire lower legs and feet. You'll start at the feet and work up until you reach the knees.

1. Use the rod to make vibrational impacts along the following:

   • Heel (direct your impact in the direction of the axis of the foot)

- Big toe (direct your impact in the direction of the axis of the foot)
- Outer edge
- Outer and inner malleoli

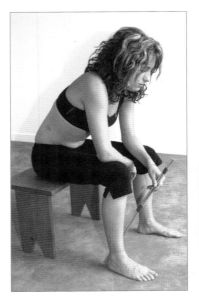 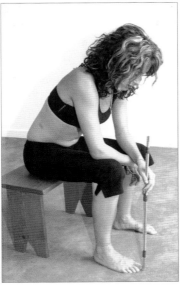 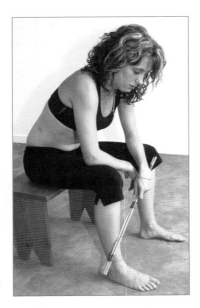

2. Work your way up the ridge of the tibia, one level at a time, until you reach the knee. The femur is generally too deep below the skin for any effective impact to be made upon it directly. You can work this bone by making an impact on the front of the knee.

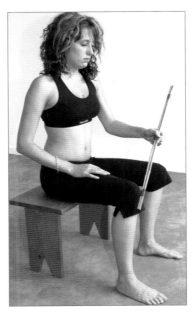

Exercises Using Scratching, Sliding, and Rubbing with Rods

It is worthwhile to work directly on the skin in order to awaken it.

The Skull and Face

This involves very gentle work that seeks to awaken awareness (sensations, feelings) of and thus the energy in this space, which over the years tends to become lifeless and unenergetic.

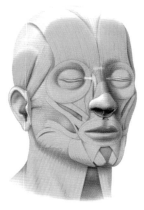

1. Explore the skull in any way your fancy takes you. Scratch the scalp area.
2. Begin the massage of your face on the forehead, moving in the direction of the jaw and with the intention of getting to know the muscles. Following the direction of the muscles, press just lightly enough to contact the muscles.
3. To massage the face with the intention of apprehending the skin, you can proceed however you wish! You may choose to follow the direction of the muscles. Use the weakest possible pressure (that of the weight of the rod).

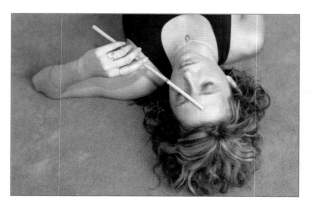
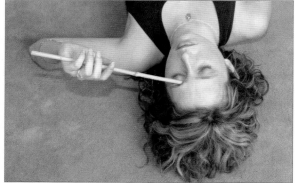

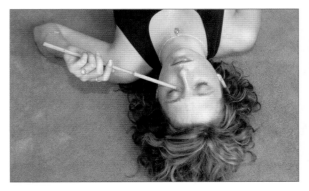
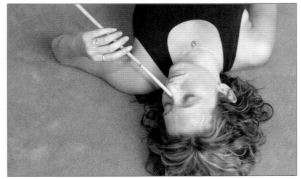
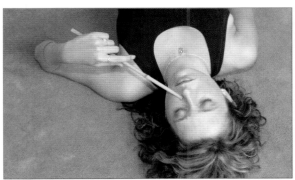
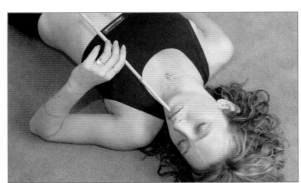

The Chest and Thorax

Start at the sternum, and work in a direction that will let you end at the tip of the shoulder and the top of the arm. This zone is very sensitive, emotionally speaking. Go over it very gently, in a state of total receptivity. Women may wish to linger here, working over their entire breast area, still very gently but affectionately.

The Upper Limbs

Your excursion in this landscape is entirely unrestricted. Each person may wander however he or she likes. You are free in accordance with your desire to follow a direction that corresponds to a particular body system: blood circulation, energy meridians, muscle direction, and so forth.

Find the position that requires the least muscular exertion in order to facilitate your receptivity.

When working on your hands, I suggest that you finish at the very tips of your fingers.

The Belly

Here too you can wander without any restriction. Again, find a position that requires the least possible muscular effort of your arm.

The Pelvis and Lower Limbs

Assume the same lying-down positions used in the vibrational exercises (see pages 140–41), and any others that best suit you.

When working on the feet, I suggest that you end at the very tips of the toes.

Other Possibilities

This book does not present every possibility for working on harmonizing the mind-body in this way, nor all the refinements that can be developed in this form of self-massage, because they require an implementation that is difficult to fully explain through word and photo.

If you delve more deeply into this kind of bodywork, you will discover on your own the adjustments you need to make for the most comfortable (and therefore most effective) positions. You will discover uses and combinations of objects that will allow you to contact even more areas with greater precision and comfort.

Comfort is important because it allows you to perform these movements without undue exertion or fatigue and therefore facilitates the receptivity and letting go necessary to achieve the full results of this practice.

Keep in mind that the tools and the techniques are not ends in themselves but simply means for helping you move about the "countryside" in a way that allows you to feel it and truly inhabit it. Beyond purely mechanical actions and beneficial reflexes, the real intention of this work has a much broader goal: to let you inhabit your life space!

12 • PRACTICAL PROTOCOLS

The practical section we are about to embark upon is designed in the spirit of the rest of this book: it is not meant to simply offer you a list of recipes but seeks to offer some practical and concrete methods you can use to relieve pain and manage some of the most common problems that affect our health and well-being. What makes this practice different from other therapeutic methods is that its methods are intended to be used within the context of a greater holistic awareness of yourself.

It is becoming more and more difficult to maintain a state of overall health. Supplements, diet, massage, essential oils, acupuncture, osteopathy, and so on—all need to be integrated into a general understanding of how your health functions, within a holistic approach of receptivity and openness to a steady stream of new discoveries about your body and yourself. These various therapies and substances should be viewed as tools that help the wheel turn more easily and move forward. Without the initial "grease" of knowledge and holistic receptivity, the wheel will come to an abrupt halt, and you will be disappointed in the results of whichever remedy you chose to restore or maintain your health.

We should look at all these healing traditions and methods as so many instruments in an orchestra when the conductor is absent. Without the conductor, the symphony runs the risk of coming to a premature end and providing disappointing results.

Pain Relief

Pain is a huge subject that I cannot claim to treat exhaustively in this book. What I focus on particularly here are the joint and muscle pains that have increasingly become the lot of everyone and are appearing in people at younger ages than ever before. Here I would like to make some clarifications.

147

Pain is not a sensation in the strict sense of the word; it is an emotion. Several factors on different levels positively or negatively influence how the pain is experienced. These factors can be related to the skin, muscles, viscera, climate, hormones, mind, or emotions.

It is possible and at times essential to remove pain, but the real question to answer is, What is behind it? What is its source? Even when the immediate problem is solved and pain may no longer be an issue, the cause persists (we can see this easily in the use of analgesics and anti-inflammatory medications). This is something I have had a lot of experience with personally in my daily practice with patients who have come to me because they are sick and tired of taking "tons and tons" of medications.

When you are told that your osteoarthritis is the problem and your X-ray is shown to you as proof, a cause-and-effect relationship is being established that is not objective. Every therapist or doctor who has any extensive experience with the subject has observed among his or her patients that there are those who suffer without any basis for it appearing on their X-rays, and, conversely, there are those who have "incriminating X-rays" but do not experience any problems.

Painful areas are those zones where the tissue and the muscles in particular are in a state of hypertonicity; this causes excess pressure and joint stiffness that is harmful to the balance of the joints and their cartilage. When the muscles are made to stop "spasming," then the pain vanishes. Of course there are also certain cases of nerve-mediated pain, such as a herniated disk, in which the core of the disk has pushed out and is mechanically compressing the nerve.

You should keep in mind one fundamental notion: the causes of pain generally include a number of factors. Among them we often find primary muscular factors that are some distance removed from the spot where the person feels pain. These places are often located in the feet and legs or the neck and head. These zones, therefore, need to be worked systematically.

Behind the pain, whether its nature is inflammatory or not, there is always a fatigue, a substantial amount of muscular tension, whatever its origin might be (primary or secondary) and whether its influence is horizontal or vertical. Everything that helps lower the tension here will contribute to relieving the pain.

The general protocol for treating pain is to work both locally and comprehensively.

Working Locally

You have already grasped the intention we will have in working directly upon a painful spot. I am going to revisit this whole notion of a "stroll in the countryside" in greater detail. Find the spot that hurts with a finger; this is the area that I suggest you work with the most delicacy. Your work with the ball or roller may also have shown you, through pain, a zone of tension of which you had been unaware.

Refer back to the discussion of bioharmony in chapter 7, so that you can allow your intention to permeate fully throughout. There is always a desire to escape tension and pain by fleeing, by moving.

Focus on the painful zone and look for the core of the contraction where it hurts most. If you are able to get inside this core, a change will occur without any effort or will required. In the beginning, the sensation of pain will intensify, due to your more acute awareness of it, but if you continue to maintain a receptive attitude and objective observation, this intensification will give way to a lessening of the pain, which will then vanish entirely. Another pain or tension may then appear. Continue to work in this same way with each new occurrence. Regard these new appearances as a positive trend, and like unwinding a tangled thread, you can follow them to a harmonizing effect. If you are not able to do this, it is most likely because the sensation is intolerable because it is connected with an unconscious psychological and emotional aspect that has been repressed.

Working Comprehensively

Working comprehensively in this context means working on the related muscle or joint chains, working both above and below the core area and concentrating your attention on the "entrances and exits," which are your hands, feet, neck, and head. It is also important to open your receptivity to the visceral area, as the organs here can exert an influence from a distance, and particularly for pains in the lumbar region.

Note: If you are dealing with a crisis involving inflammation, lumbago, or a hyperalgesiac zone, I suggest you avoid working on that area directly. Instead, concentrate on a spot at a distance, working on the "exits" and the ends of the muscle chains.

We are going to look at the most common pains next, but the protocol is the same for other pains. It is valuable to know which muscle is involved and which chains it belongs to, to devote attention both upstream and downstream of it, and to work on the exits (particularly toward the feet).

The pain and the tension is unique for each individual depending on the factors that are an influence (causes). Something that might work well for one person will not necessarily work well for someone else. But the time you take for yourself, in this approach and in this intention, will always be beneficial for you.

When addressing pains, I advise you to adopt whenever possible a prone position (or else end the session in one), because it is the most naturally relaxing.

You should spend several minutes working on each zone, or more if you feel the need. Your choice of tools and place are all a matter of time, your desire, and what feels right. Simply respect the broad guidelines provided by this book. I will provide several protocols by way of suggestion.

Head

I can suggest two different "excursions" here: one using the roller and ball, and one using the rod in the vibrational technique.

With the Roller and Ball

1. Use the roller beneath your head.
2. Use the ball beneath the base of the skull and behind the neck.
3. Use the roller behind the lumbar area and the sacrum.

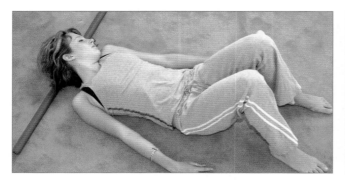
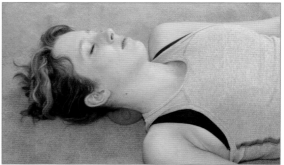
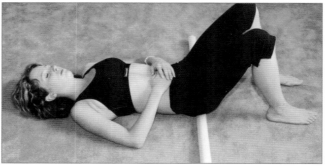

4. Continue with the roller beneath the calf, behind the Achilles' tendon, and under the heel.

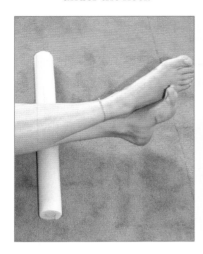 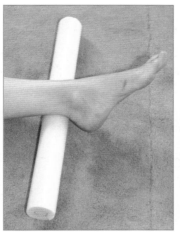 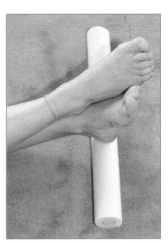

5. End with the feet.

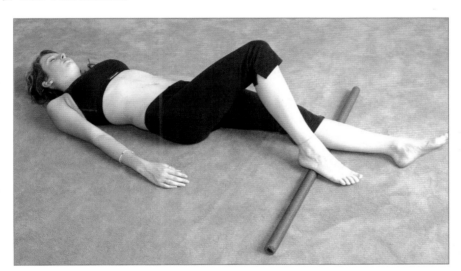

With the Rod

1. Use the vibrational technique with the rods at head level.
2. Work with the rods at the level of the arms, including the shoulders, clavicle, and thorax.
3. End the session by working the Achilles' tendon, heels, and feet.

Cervicalgia

Cervicalgia is a condition of frequently occurring neck pain that does not radiate outward. Whether or not an X-ray provides evidence of osteoarthritis, the treatment involves working on the muscle contractions. Massage the region locally, then work on the nearest "exits." You can use the same roller-and-ball protocol just described for the head, placing emphasis on the neck and the base of the skull.

Cervicobrachial Neuralgia

The protocol for cervicobrachial neuralgia, or sciatica of the arm, is the same as for cervicalgia. Establish contact with the neck and the base of the skull for the local massage. Here your emphasis should be on opening the arms, and you should finish this session working on the Achilles' tendon, heels, and feet.

Pain in the Trapezius

The trapezius muscle, rising over the inside tip of the shoulder blade, is often a source of pain, typically stress related. To address it, work with a ball behind the spine at the level of the shoulder blade. Bring the ball up the spine to the major source of pain, which is where the trapezius muscle connects to the base of the skull. Continue working the ball down the back of the shoulder blade and then down the arms, all the way to the hands.

Shoulder Pain

The shoulders are the crossroads between the arms and the axis of the body. I suggest that you put your intention to opening the arm and neck, working toward the back and the lower half of the body.

Elbow Pain

In many cases elbow pain has an important primary origin in the neck area. Look to open the neck and the forearm.

Lumbar Pain

Who hasn't experienced lumbar pain, either acute or chronic? It afflicts people at younger and younger ages now. The lumbar zone absorbs a lot of pressures, burdens, and blocks connected with the basal dimensions of our personal history. This zone requires exploration on a regular basis, even when it is not truly painful.

Here are two protocols:

- While lying down, work with the roller beneath the head, behind the lumbar spine, behind the sacrum at two or three different levels, and under the calves, the Achilles' tendons, the heels, and then the feet.
- While standing, explore the back surface of your entire torso, using either a roller or a ball, down to the sacrum. End this session with work on your Achilles' tendons, heels, and feet.

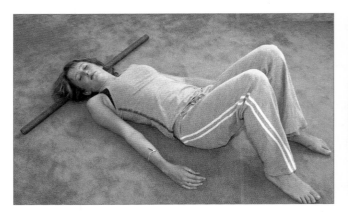
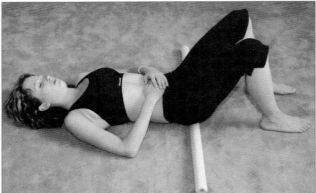

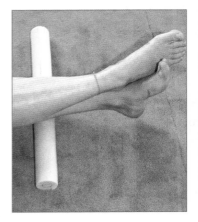
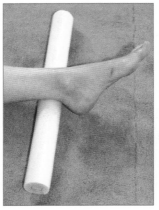
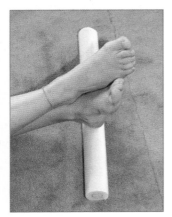

Lumbago

Lumbago is almost always triggered by a little gesture, the last straw . . . a trifle (a reflexive movement that regularly goes unnoticed) can cause it—with very spectacular symptoms. Force yourself to keep moving and resist the temptation to stay still.

I suggest that you work below the painful area, toward the pelvis and lower limbs. End with work on the Achilles' tendons and heels.

Sciatica

It should be noted that pains mimicking sciatica are much more frequent than true sciatica. In fact, herniated disks have been found to be present in 20 to 30 percent of people presenting no symptoms. They cannot be blamed willy-nilly for causing sciatic pain. But in the rare cases where they are truly the cause of this pain, you should still ask yourself what the true origin of the pain might be. It could involve muscle spasms compressing the spinal column on one side, causing the ejection of the disk and potential irritation of the sciatic nerve (true sciatica).

Releasing Tensions, Relaxing, and Decompressing

All these acts are interrelated!

There are countless relaxation techniques. Some can make you feel as if you are soaring or floating; some guide you on splendid journeys through beautiful landscapes; some cause you to no longer feel your body. But that is not the approach here. What we are seeking to do instead is to anchor ourselves, embody our awareness, and truly inhabit it. The results of this approach are the easing of the muscles, true relaxation, and relief of mind and body.

Refer back to the discussion of bioharmony in chapter 7 so that you clearly grasp the intention and spirit of this approach. The protocol to use for this work is the same as that used for treating pain. In fact, all the exercises offered in this book are going to help you relax, decompress, and let go of your tensions. The basic protocol is always valid and can be the basis for countless combinations.

My suggestion here would be to use the roller and to create a broad protocol of massage sequences (based on how much time you have, your feelings, and what you desire) that includes your head, neck, upper limbs, torso, lower limbs, and feet, working from top to bottom.

Here are several suggestions:

- While lying down, work with the roller from your head to your feet.
- While standing, work the upper limbs, then work down from your head to your sacrum. Lie down to finish by working on your legs and feet.
- Do all the vibration exercises, starting at your head and working down to your feet.

Reducing Stress Levels

Everyone is in agreement that life has become more stressful, and stress is the chief source of feeling physically and psychologically run down. Stress is the body's response to situations that require rapid and effective adaptation to the demands of our environment. In our modern society, with all its constraints and demands, various forms of pollution, the pace of life, pressures, and so on, we may find it increasingly difficult to manage and maintain our stress reactions within boundaries that will not cause problems for our bodies and damage our overall health.

Without going into the details, there are three major types of strategies for reducing stress. One of these is more particularly worthwhile for us than the others. It is centered on the reduction of the stress reaction and the increase of our resistance to it; it relies on relaxation techniques to work.

Under this word *relaxation* are grouped together a set of techniques whose purpose is to obtain the weakest level of muscular tension possible, accompanied by a sense of psychological relief, while maintaining the mind in an alert state of awareness (the official definition, if I may put it that way).

This relief state, also known as the relaxation response, can be defined as the opposite of the stress reaction, encompassing a slowdown of heart rate and breathing and a reduction of muscle tone, blood pressure, adrenaline rate, and limbic system activity.

The self-massage work that is the subject of this book is a very effective and practical tool for initiating the relaxation response. Every little excursion you make across your body will be highly profitable. Focus on the zones that you feel are stretched, overburdened, or painful, or simply those that you wish to work.

The roller is the preferred tool for these massages, as it allows you to make contact with large surface areas and to apply stronger pressure. You should work lying down, if possible, and always end the session with work on your legs and feet. Opening the lower limbs and feet is always of great benefit, no matter what problem you are working on. It summons our energy and awareness into the lower half of our body, when generally our energy and awareness have a tendency to get settled in our upper half.

The general protocol is to start at head level and work downward, ending with the lower limbs and feet. You should pass over both the upper limbs and the torso, but it is always your choice which zones you wish to focus on. For example, you could:

- Work with the roller beneath the base of your skull and then, in succession, the shoulder, elbow, wrist, sacrum, Achilles' tendon, and heel.
- Work the head, the spinal column, the legs, and the feet.

Clear Your Head and Calm Your Mind

The ideal protocol for clearing your head would be to get away for an entire week from your daily routine! Lacking this, these relaxation techniques and self-massages can be quite profitable.

The general protocol is always the same: start by working on your head (you can choose which tool you prefer; experiment!), then work on the zone that feels overburdened, tense, or painful. Go over your upper limbs in stages from shoulder to hand, and end with your legs and feet. For example, you could:

- Work with the rod on your face and skull, and then use a roller to work on your elbows, hands, legs, and feet.
- While standing, work on your face and skull, then do the entire back in successive stages down to the sacrum. Lie down to finish your self-massage session by working on your feet and legs with the rollers.

There are many possibilities, depending on your preferences and the time you have at your disposal. Always save some time to devote to opening your awareness in your legs and feet.

Relief of Swollen and Bloated Stomach

I meet many people who complain of feeling bloated all the time despite eating a balanced diet. Diet has nothing to do with it. In reality, this bloating is the result of stress caused by a burden or inner tension that cannot resolve itself and therefore cannot be "digested" and "evacuated." All body and mind work that promotes relaxation and letting go will allow you to release this burden. For this kind of self-massage I suggest you use the deep draining of the stomach (see page 104) combined with work on the lower limbs (see page 109).

Relief of Heavy and Swollen Legs

Here is a problem that affects many people, particularly women. The factors involved are many, in unique proportions for every individual. Often standard medical examinations will reveal poor circulation due to problems with the blood or lymph vessels. Among the other factors, one that is not often mentioned but that can contribute, sometimes significantly, to the severity of the disorder is muscle tension.

As veins travel between the muscles, the muscle fasciae and their excessive tension can constrict the vessels. All work that reduces muscular tension will contribute to improving the situation and also serve as a maintenance measure. Self-massages are the tool of choice here, as they will act upon the muscles by easing their tone and mechanically assist the flow of circulation.

All the tools offered in this practice will provide positive benefits. Two methods in particular can be very productive:

- Working the back of the legs, especially the soleus muscle (the muscle behind the calf muscle); this is a highly stimulating muscle through which many blood vessels travel.
- Vibration work on the lower limbs, especially when you lie on your back with your legs raised against a wall.

Here is the protocol for vibration work on the lower limbs:

1. Lie on your back with your legs propped up against a wall. To position yourself properly, with your heels and buttocks pressed against the wall, it's easiest to first lie on your side with your legs next to the wall, then pivot your legs and torso to achieve the desired position.

2. With the help of a rod, begin creating vibrations from the bony points on your foot and up along the ridge of the tibia until you reach the knee.

3. When you reach the knee, which should be slightly flexed, lightly flick the knee first upward (directing your impact and its vibrations in the direction of the tibia) and then downward (directing your impact and its vibrations in the direction of the femur).

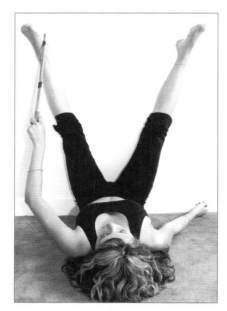
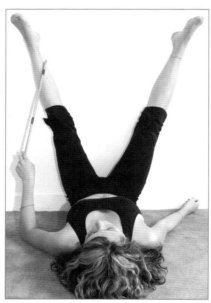

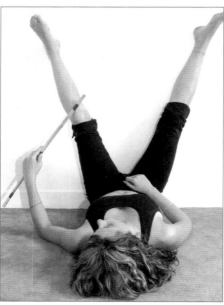

Note: You can also use the vibration technique on your skin and muscles from your feet down to the top of your thighs.

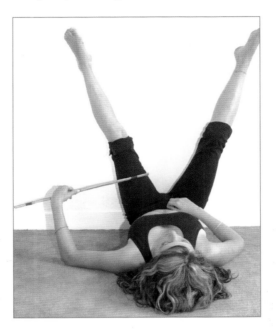

Grounding Ourselves

We can't deny that our modern life is separating us more and more from the ground, the earth. Every day we are compelled to reflect, project, anticipate, foresee, protect, and defend ourselves, living like this some five feet above the ground. This hyperactivity on the mental level costs us dearly. We pay for it with mental and emotional tensions that congest in our upper half and empty our bottom half.

Anything that can concretely call up, awaken, and help circulate energy and awareness through the lower half of the body facilitates a flow of life toward the bottom and draws forth the energy of that area, which in turn will help decongest the top.

Note: Freeing the top facilitates a flow toward the bottom, but this is not always enough, as the top can rapidly become corked up again. Nor is opening receptivity in the lower half of your body always sufficient. In reality, everything that allows you to open up and relax, no matter where in the body it takes place, will help you feel more levelheaded and steady.

Increasing Body Awareness

Among the various means for awakening the consciousness of the body, bioharmonic self-massage offers multiple "discovery-filled excursions" for rediscovering your body and learning how to inhabit your most intimate living space. Each exploration you undertake will reconnect you a little more, and make you feel more as one. This holistic mind-body work contributes to a sensation of oneness.

Discover your skin with the rods or the foam ball; discover your bones through the vibration techniques; and so on with your flesh, your organs . . .

Self-Massage through Meditation

Numerous forms of meditation rely on different forms of physical support, which provides self-massage. This kind of meditation allows you to calm your mind and to feel as one—to experience the disappearance of the duality between the observer and the thing observed.

Inner Seeking

This approach offers the finishing touch to psychological work by facilitating the cleansing of the emotional charge created by any unresolved issue. As you now realize, the psycho-emotional dimension is always imprinted within the very tissue of our bodies.

We think we are relaxed because we are not feeling any pain; we need to quit fooling ourselves! When we take time to listen to ourselves and tune in, whether through yoga, massage, or any other means, our consciousness awakens and we discover that in reality we are not as relaxed as we had thought. Our consciousness was simply too superficial. This realization is often cause for astonishment. After massaging one of their arms, or a shoulder, people have often told me, "I thought I was completely relaxed and then I realized I actually was far from it!"

Through my own personal and professional experience, one thing has become increasingly clear: the mental and emotional dimension of our own histories leaves a deep imprint in our bodily tissue. Making conscious contact with this tissue is equivalent to a deep cleansing—working through the deep and fundamental causes of our disharmony, or our dysfunctions.

The body is emotional—and emotion is corporeal!

Many mind-body approaches concentrate on the relationship of the mind with the body and the role it plays in healing the body. But there is another way to look at the relationship of the body with the mind, one that studies the role of the body in healing. In the bioharmonic approach, instead of asking what thought, feeling, or emotion is affecting the body, we explore the way in which a specific sensation helps us to understand and connect with an emotional or psychological problem.

To really heal and restore ourselves, we need to root our emotional experience inside our bodies and unearth the emotional and psychological problems behind our physical sensations. In all cases, the body is the fulcrum for this work. Concretely, if you are already in one form of psychotherapy or another, this self-massage body-mind work can be truly beneficial. It facilitates realization and the full integration of the traumatic event by the liberation of the emotional burden encoded inside the body. This work by itself is much harder, requiring you to be really "plugged in" to your emotional being.

Pick a part of your body on which you are going to work. There are two ways in which you can do this:

- Spontaneously choose a painful or tense zone or, quite simply, the one that most draws your attention or most interests you. Now, open your intention to establish contact with every emotion, thought, or image that seems to have a deep connection and resonance with this zone.
- Focus your awareness on the emotion, thought, or problem that is most important in your life right now, and spontaneously put a finger on the part of your body that seems the most connected and resonant with it.

Touch this part of your body with the help of a ball or roller. Bring your attention to the physical sensation present there (and express in words what this sensation feels like to you), without trying to change, control, or analyze this zone. During this process, you might have sensations—thoughts, emotions, images, colors, and so on—that appear elsewhere and start interfering with your attention. Note their presence but do not follow them, keeping your awareness on the physical sensation at the place you are touching. If this sensation changes, follow the new sensation that has emerged. From time to time, clarify what you are experiencing by verbalizing it. Take ten to fifteen minutes to perform this exercise.

By concentrating on the physical sensation rather than the emotional problems connected to it, you allows these emotions to come to the surface and transform.

For example, a person is aware of a tension in her shoulder and the anger that is attached to it. If she concentrates on this anger, she could bring back to mind the incident that triggered it and generate even more tension and anger (this is sometimes useful and necessary, though). However, it is possible that this anger may conceal a deeper emotion. If she concentrates on her sensations, she may observe her anger rising. If she remains present at the spot of tension, sorrow might emerge from where the anger was, and she may experience trembling where the pain had been. If she remains in this deeply receptive awareness of the trembling sensation, solitude, for example, may replace the sorrow and relaxation take the place of the trembling. The process could end here. Or it could continue, and she may attain a state where the tensions become unknotted. The sensation and the emotional problem melt into each other and disappear. In all cases, the person has the sensation that something has gone, that the corporeal space is open and a little more inhabited.

Ancient Wisdom and Modern Thought

The following conviction can be found in Buddhism: if you concentrate long enough on an emotion, you shall attain the corporeal sensation hiding behind it. If you concentrate long enough on the corporeal sensation, you shall attain the biochemical reactions that produce this sensation. If you concentrate long enough on these biochemical reactions, you shall attain the molecular components that gave birth to them. And if you concentrate long enough on the molecular components, you shall attain the most fundamental particles, called *kalapas*, which cannot be divided.

Kalapas are said to resemble solid particles. In fact they are waves of vibration. According to Buddhist thought, vibrational energy is the fundamental reality. Sensation and emotion arise out of this fundamental unity. And it is back into this fundamental unity that they dissolve.

When we identify ourselves with a sensation and a feeling, we identify ourselves with our suffering. When we go back toward that unity by accompanying the sensation and the feeling, we move out of suffering into healing.

This notion, discovered 2,500 years ago, has resurfaced in modern physics, which essentially reveals that the fundamental particles are not solid but made up of vibrational waves. Both ancient wisdom and modern thought have reached the same conclusion: the fundamental reality is not a mass of separate entities but a unified vibrational field. Our ordinary experience—thoughts, feelings, sensations—emerges out of this fundamental unity and can return and become one with it.

Healing is unity. The two words *healing* and *wholeness* share a common ancestor, the Old English word *hael*. This word is also the root for the words *holy* and *hallowed*. This is how compassion becomes linked with the sacred and spirituality. In order to heal, we need this sacred foundation of healing.

Face Lifting

This is a natural technique that requires no plastic surgery or miracle cream! Look at a little child. His face, skin, muscles, and tissue are still full of life, energy, and openness. Now look at our adult faces and touch their skin. It is a little loose and slack. Look at those double and triple chins, the pouches, pits, and lumps that took shape as time passed. We tell ourselves that our skin is just aging. That's true enough, but a more important cause of this degeneration is withdrawal of energy and awareness from our skin as life goes by and we experience blows, traumas, and other various psycho-emotional tensions.

When we inhabit our face again and reconnect with it in awareness and sensation, our skin and muscle will naturally contribute to restoring tone to the inner tissue. This is not a miracle technique; all it requires is that we regularly devote a little time to massaging it every day, just as we wash and groom ourselves.

Work on the skin of the face with the tip of a wand, applying the gentlest pressure, just enough to let you feel the thickness of the skin.

Self-Massage and Bioenergetic Resynchronization

Changes in the body's energy circulation system cannot be separated from changes in muscle tone and other physical and physiological changes.

Wherever you place your consciousness (sensations, feelings), your energy will be. When you take time to tune in to yourself, each time you inhabit your body with awareness, it is energy that sets up shop there.

You can use these self-massages with the intention of stimulating acupoints and energy meridian but also to feel this vibrational aspect, these impulses, waves, and currents (everyone perceives them in their own fashion). This is a tricky world to handle. Be careful that you don't "take off" and start flying.

Other Applications

Other applications are possible—it is up to you to discover them. My intention is not to offer you some kind of panacea with a book of recipes, nor to promote these self-massages to you as the best possible technique. Like all others, this approach has its advantages, as well as its drawbacks and limitations. In this first book on the subject, I have presented you with a tool that is rich with practical applications. These self-massages are a pretext for rehabilitating your body and reconciling with it—and therefore with yourself.

CONCLUSION

You have now reached the end of this book, and, perhaps, you have lingered over the exercises and left the theoretical and critical first half to read later. It appeared important to me as I wrote this book not merely to give you techniques but to encourage you to reflect and expand your awareness concerning this field of health and the body-mind relationship.

I addressed your left brain (analytical, rational) through the sciences, and I addressed your right brain as well, so that when you finished reading this book, something would have changed inside of you, in the way you look at things, in your understanding, and in your behavior. Grasping something intellectually is always worthwhile. But if nothing changes in our actions . . .

In the first part of the book I tried to share with you, supported by scientific proofs, a more holistic and unified vision of how we function. This better understanding of the different dimensions of the human being and their synergy allows us to reconcile, in a complementary and constructive way, the many existing therapies, in order to see that each approach has something to contribute to this infinite interactive puzzle. It opens new fields for exploration and provides new grounds for hope.

In the several decades that have elapsed while I have been training, experimenting, and learning more about this domain, I realized the extent to which, when a person becomes a specialist, he or she insidiously and quickly adopts a distorted perspective. A specialist can become sectarian, seeing things only through the lens of his or her own approach and forgetting or renouncing what he or she once loved. Of course, it takes all kinds to make a world. Each of us hears what we are ready to hear, and in my work I have learned and am still learning to respect the expectations of other individuals and not impose my point of view on others. I have also realized that many people are ready to open up and are just waiting for the opportunity, not knowing where to find the information they need, or even completely unaware that so many other possibilities even exist.

The more you know, the less you know. You think you have identified a problem, and you then discover other ramifications, other connections. You think you have performed a real feat, and then practice shows you that things are a bit more nuanced. The further you advance into this landscape and the more you discover, the more you realize the infinite perspectives that are possible. You realize that it is endless and relative, and therefore full of hope and potential, because nothing is fixed and frozen.

We are all quite ignorant, even we specialists. We have ready-made ideas, established beliefs in many different fields, most particularly the one that interests us personally. I am struck by the fact that despite the scientific evidence, the objective knowledge, and concrete cases, there are many who turn a deaf ear and don't want to challenge in any way the edifice on which they are enthroned.

Disinformation, noninformation, single-mindedness or fixated thoughts, all our beliefs and well-rooted ideas, sustained by different and varied shades of self-interest, make it so we are moving through a flood of all kinds of pressures, fears, and insecurities. This makes it hard for us to stop by the edge of the path to contemplate the expanse of the landscape and be open to it. It makes it hard for us to become truly informed and discover all that is serious and objective, even if it sometimes appears absolutely insane and totally opposed to the dominant trends.

The majority of significant scientific advances have been made by seekers who had the courage to ask the questions that loomed up following their observation of phenomena that didn't "fit" into the framework of existing theory. The best known is Copernicus, who had the courage to totally change his starting hypothesis explaining the movement of the planets of the solar system. Instead of believing that the old theory was correct at 90 percent, he told himself that if 10 percent of the phenomena observed did not fit into the theory's framework, then it was entirely false.

There have been many other scientific advances that have revolutionized physics, such as quantum mechanics, for one example. We are compelled to acknowledge that all these seekers, whatever century they lived in, experienced a lot of trouble because they called back into question too many habits and vested interests.

In the field of health and medicine, the theories and works of Dr. Hamer* are one example. They represent a quantum leap in contemporary medical thought. They represent a veritable "Copernican revolution" in the understanding of illness.

Short and sweet! This is how we envision successful medical intervention: that it shouldn't require any effort or personal involvement, thanks to a multitude of easy methods to which we hold out our hands.

So much information and so many new methodologies and tools are invading the health market today that we risk getting lost, hopping from one thing to the next, maneuvering between Scylla and Charybdis, as we leave allopathy to throw ourselves into the arms of homeopathy, acupuncture, osteopathy, massage therapies, and so forth, without understanding their mechanisms or the synergies and processes they put in play for maintaining health and balance. Yet all these therapies, even if they tend to be more natural processes, remain simply crutches.

I have met many people in my practice who go shopping all the time at the market of therapeutic consumption. They have not grasped that it is not the tool that cures but themselves. All these techniques they have tested, the lectures they've attended, and the workshops they've taken have been absorbed in the consciousness that healing is something outside the self, and that it is the other person and his technique that are doing the healing. Health care is not provided by the will but with letting go, receptiveness, and love of yourself.

Through these self-massages and this book, I have tried to contribute my own little piece to your well-being. I hope that beyond the tools and techniques I've brought you, I have aroused your curiosity and expanded your understanding and the way you look at your physical reality; at the synergy between your body, energies, sensations, emotions, brain, and consciousness; and at the potential for well-being that opening your body consciousness can bring you. I hope I have opened the horizon for you in the way you envision things, the way you understand your problems, and the way you take action.

---

*Dr. Hamer is currently jailed in France for advising cancer patients in alternatives to standard treatments. His studies of brain scans have revealed that each physical trauma has a corresponding location in the brain.

I do not know if "the voices of the Lord are impenetrable," but I do know that there are many, some of which have yet to come, and others of which I am unaware or that I do not even suspect exist. When you decide to take yourself in hand and expand your quest beyond the beaten paths, you will open the doors of understanding and hope and give yourself new potential for health and well-being.

The ascent of man into heaven is not the key, but rather his ascent here into the spirit and the descent also of the spirit into his normal humanity and the transformation of this earthly nature. For that and not some post mortem salvation is the real new birth for which humanity waits as the crowning movement of its long, obscure and painful course. An immense spiritual revolution that rehabilitates Matter and the creation. One can say that it is when the circle is truly completed and the two opposites are joined, when the highest manifests in the most physical—the supreme Reality in the heart of the atom— that the experience will reach its true conclusion. It seems that one never really understands unless one understands with one's body.

THE MOTHER'S AGENDA

APPENDIX I • MATTER VERSUS MIND

This line indicates the demarcation between the "outside" of space-time (located above the line) and the "inside" of space-time (located below the line).

Everything that is above the line of demarcation is visible and more generally accessible by our sense organs.

Everything that is below the line of demarcation is directly accessible to the mind but only indirectly accessible to our sense organs.

On either side of the line there is thus a different "substance." One is notably visible; the other is not. The first should be defined as matter and the other Mind. These two substances have no direct interaction; in other words, an object that is located below cannot go above and "collide," for example, with an object above. But indirect interactions, that is to say with no exchange of objects, can exist between the objects on either side of the line. These indirect exchanges (which physicists call, following Feynmann's lead, "virtual" interactions) are comparable to what happens when you see yourself in a mirror. You cannot enter the space that is behind the mirror, as it is a virtual world. However, you see that if you lift your arm, your virtual image in the mirror also lifts his or her arm. There is therefore an indirect influence between your world and the virtual world appearing in the mirror.

The atomic nucleus, which when enlarged 1,000 billion times would (for carbon) be a pile of twelve balls forming a sphere around 1 centimeter in diameter, should be represented in the "outside" of space-time (which is to say above the line of demarcation). The electron (about 1 or 2 millimeters in diameter in our example), to the contrary, would be located beneath the line of demarcation, and therefore geometrically represented with *nonzero* dimensions in the "inside" of space-time. But seen from the outside of space-time, which is to say directly grasped by our sense organs, the electron leaves only a trace of its point of contact with the line of demarcation, and so it thus appears as an object "without volume," and more generally without any definable geometrical shape. In short it is invisible in the "inside" of space-time. It is an object that can be directly grasped only by the mind. In fact, *it is Mind;* whereas the protons and neutrons are *Matter.*

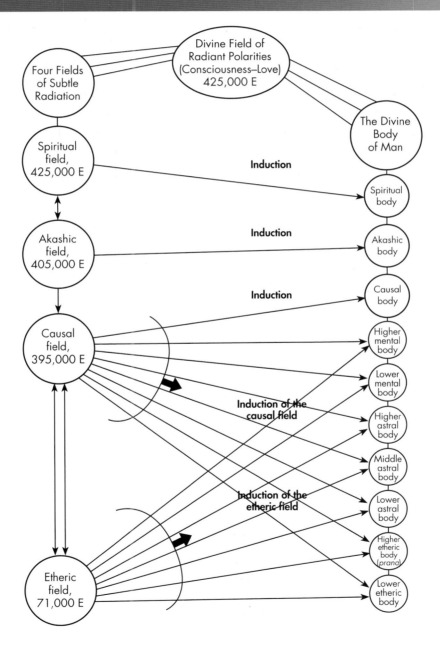

APPENDIX III • THE SEVEN RINGS OF BODY ARMOR

Here is how Wilhelm Reich describes the seven rings of body armor (or the seven breastplates) in his book *Character Analysis*.

The **ocular armor ring** includes the forehead, the eyes, the tear ducts, and the region of the malar bones. This ring hides within its emotional expression terror, panic, anguish, emptiness, the inability to weep, the refusal to see or express emotions through the eyes, the inability to look someone in the eyes, and all the ocular problems related to myopia, strabismus, and so on. It is the first armor ring to appear after birth, once the child starts seeking to connect with life outside his mother's womb through his eyes.

The **oral armor ring** includes the chin muscles, the lips, the throat, and the back of the head (occiput). This ring conceals the desire to cry, to suck, to bite, to vociferate, to grimace, and all the emotions connected to these activities. The second armor ring to develop, it is associated with the first year of the nursing infant's life, from when it begins breastfeeding until it begins eating solid food, and it corresponds to the expression of the child's first needs of hunger and thirst. This ring conceals the emotions connected to deep sorrow, boredom, despair, anger, and frustration.

The **neck armor ring** includes the deep muscles of the neck and tongue. This armor ring hides in its emotional expression the restraint of emotions, tears, anger, and the reflex of "swallowing" one's feelings. It is the third piece of body armor to develop and corresponds to the emotional expression of the nursing child, to the child's unfulfilled communication needs, when it babbles, smiles, and establishes relations with the other.

The **chest armor ring** includes the thorax and its muscles (intercostals, pectorals, and deltoids), the organs of the chest (lungs and heart), and the muscles of the arms. This armor hides cardiac problems, anxiety, reserve, self-control, holding back, constraint, immobility, awkwardness with the normally expressive movements of the arms and hands, hardheartedness, stiff-neckedness, inaccessibility, indifference, and the inability to take. The emotions related to this armor are deep sorrow, despair, anguish, tears, rage, and the impression of having a knot in one's chest. It is the fourth segment to develop and corresponds to the years when the child experiences the traumatizing memory of bad treatment, disappointment, loss, abandonment, and rejection. Wilhelm regarded this segment as the core of the armoring, as it is the central piece.

The **diaphragmatic armor ring** includes the diaphragm and its organs (liver, gallbladder, stomach, pancreas, and spleen). This armor includes in its affective expression the desire to defend against the sensations of anxiety and pleasure, feeling cut in two, and the separation from the top and the bottom. It is formed at a later age, and its development is connected to the first experiences of the pleasurable waves that emanate from the pelvis and genitals.

The **abdominal armor ring** includes the abdominal muscles, the transverse and psoas muscles, and the square of the loins, the entrails, the kidneys, and the adrenal glands. It is constructed at the same age as the diaphragmatic and pelvic rings and is connected to the refusal to experience pleasure, feelings of emptiness, and the need for control of life, to hold on to things and not expel them, to be clean to meet one's parents' needs, compulsive behavior, fear, the cutting of the umbilical cord, and separation anxiety.

The **pelvic armor ring** includes all the muscles of the pelvis, the genital organs, the anus, the perineum, and the muscles of the legs. Its affective expression includes asexuality, anger, anxiety, destructive rage, despair, and sorrow. It is the last armor segment to form and it does so at the same time as the diaphragmatic and abdominal rings.

APPENDIX IV • THE NATURE OF GENERALIZATION

Generalization is the superposition of several facets of the same sign in one piece of consistent information.

Generalization should not be confused with a simple synthesis.

Synthesis tells us that the meaning that is assigned to this sign sometimes means white and sometimes means black. Now these two meanings are rendered false or incomplete as I give this sign the meaning of being gray.

Generalization tells us that this sign sometimes means white and sometimes means black. Both meanings are acceptable, because one face or facet of the sign is white and the other is black. In other words, generalization should be distinguished from synthesis in the sense that it is never the compromise between thesis and antithesis. It endeavors to show that the thesis and antithesis are both acceptable meanings, which complement each other like the opposing faces of the same sign.

For example, the cross section of a cylinder on a plane following its axis is a rectangle. When taken on a plane perpendicular to the cylinder's axis, the cross section is a circle.

The different meanings of a sign do not replace one another but complete each other to provide a more complete and harmonious spiritual representation—which is to say less contradictory—of this sign, with the reservation that successive generalizations, as many as they may be, will never attain an absolute representation of the outside world and that knowledge is a path that moves forward by expanding without ever ending.

BIBLIOGRAPHY

Alexander, Gerda. *Eutony: The Holistic Discovery of the Entire Person*. New York: Felix Morrow, 1986.

Aurobindo, Sri. *Supramental Manifestations Upon Earth*. Twin Lakes, Wis.: Lotus Press, 1949.

———. *The Synthesis of Yoga*. New York: The Sri Aurobindo Library, 1950.

Bohm, David. *Wholeness and the Implicate Order*. London: Routledge and Kegan Paul, 1981.

Bois, Danis. *Le Sensible et le mouvement*. Ivry-sur-Seine, France: Point d'appui, 2001.

Boyesen, Gerda. *Entre Psyché et soma*. Paris: Payot, 1997.

Brieghel-Müller, Gunna. *Eutony and Relaxation: The Release of Physical and Mental Tension*. Translated by Joan Deedes. United Kingdom: GBM Editions, 2004.

Brosse, Thérèse. *La Conscience-energie, structure de l'homme et de l'univers*. Paris: Editions Presence, 2003.

Brousse, Myriam. *Le corps ne le sait pas encore*. Aubagne, France: Editions Quintessence, 1998.

Charon, Jean E. *L'esprit, cet inconnu*. Paris: Albin Michel, 1977. Translated into English as *Unknown Spirit* (Sigo Press, 1983).

———. *Le tout, l'esprit et la matière*. Paris: Albin Michel, 1987.

———. *Mort, voici ta defaite*. Paris: Albin Michel, 1979.

Chopra, Deepak. *Quantum Healing*. New York: Bantam Books, 1996.

Damasio, Antonio. *Descartes' Error: Emotion, Reason, and the Human Brain*. New York, London: Penguin Books, 2005.

———. *Looking for Spinoza: Joy, Sorrow, and the Feeling Brain*. New York: Houghton Mifflin Harcourt, 2003.

De Souzenelle, Annick. *La Symbolique du corps*. Escalquens, France: Editions Dangles, 1997.

Dutheil, Régis. *L'Homme superlumineux*. Paris: Sand & Tchou, 2006.

———. *La Médicine superlumineuse*. Paris: Sand & Tchou, 1999.

Fiammetti, Roger. *Le langage émotionnel du corps*. Paris: Ed. Dervy, 2004.

Flèche, Christian, and Jean-Jacques Lagardet. *L'instant de la guérison*. Gap, France: Le Souffle d'Or, 2007.

Ford, Clyde W. *Compassionate Touch: The Body's Role in Emotional Healing and Recovery.* Berkeley, Calif.: North Atlantic, 1999.

Frogier, J. F. *Aux Sources de l'anthropologie.* Meolans-Revel, France: DesIris, 1988.

Garnier-Mallet, Jean-Pierre. *Changer votre future par les ouvertures temporelles.* Agnières, France: Le Temps Present, 2006.

Grosjean, D., and P. Benini. *Pacifier corps et mémoires.* Swiss edition in three languages—French, English, German. London: Publishing Training Centre, 1993.

Guinée, Dr. Robert. *Les maladies, mémoires de l'évolution.* Brussels, Belgium: Amyris Editions, 2004.

Hamer, Ryke Geerd. *Summary of the New Medicine.* Austria: Amici di Dirk, 2000.

Labonté, Marie-Lise. *Au Coeur de notre corps.* Quebec: Editions de l'Homme, 2000.

———. *Le déclic.* Quebec: Editions de l'Homme, 2004.

Lahy, Georges. *La voix du corps.* Lascours, France: Editions Lahy, 2005.

The Mother's Agenda. Ottawa: Institute for Evolutionary Research, 1992.

Mouret, Michel-Gabriel. *Symbolique de l'image en anthropologie.* Meolans-Revel, France: DesIris, 1996.

Odoul, Michel. *Dis-moi où tu as mal.* Paris: Albin Michel, 2002.

Painter, Jack. *Deep Bodywork and Personal Development.* Mill Valley, Calif.: Bodymind Books, 1986.

Salomon, Paule. *La femme solaire.* Paris: Albin Michel, 1991.

———. *Les homes se tranforment.* Paris: Albin Michel, 1999.

———. *La sainte folie du couple.* Paris: Albin Michel, 1994.

Satprem. *The Legend of the Future.* Ottawa: Institute for Evolutionary Research, 1999.

———. *The Mind of the Cells.* Ottawa: Institute for Evolutionary Research, 1982.

———. *The Revolt of the Earth.* Ottawa: Institute for Evolutionary Research, 1990.

———. *The Tragedy of the Earth: From Sophocles to Sri Aurobindo.* Ottawa: Institute for Evolutionary Research, 1995.

Servan-Schreiber, David. *The Instinct to Heal: Curing Stress, Anxiety, and Depression without Drugs and without Talk Therapy.* Emmaus, Penn.: Rodale Books, 2004.

Soulas, Johann. *Au délà du Coeur.* Loretteville, Quebec: Ed. Dauphin Blanc, 1999.

———. *La Conscience de l'Ordre fusionnel.* Loretteville, Quebec: Ed. Dauphin Blanc, 2000.

———. *Le couronnement de la vie.* Loretteville, Quebec: Ed. Dauphin Blanc, 1999.

———. *Éveil à la conscience universelle.* Paris: Argel, 1999.

———. *La Genèse de l'homme divin.* Loretteville, Quebec: Ed. Dauphin Blanc, 1999.

———. *L'Humanité en gestation.* Loretteville, Quebec: Ed. Dauphin Blanc, 1999.

———. *La Libération par l'éveil.* Loretteville, Quebec: Ed. Dauphin Blanc, 1999.

———. *La Synergie à l'éveil.* Loretteville, Quebec: Ed. Dauphin Blanc, 1999.

Surany, Marguerite de. *Les deux inseparables: crane-colonne.* Paris: Ed. Guy Trédaniel, 1990.

———. *Dictionnaire de la medicine taoïste.* Paris: Ed. Guy Trédaniel, 2001.

ABOUT THE AUTHOR

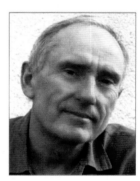

Yves Bligny has had a lifelong interest in the body as a source of balance and overall health. He is a:

- Physical education teacher
- Physical fitness trainer
- Therapist and teacher of Eutonie (at the G. Alexander School of Copenhagen)
- Kinesiology therapist and masseur trained in various forms of holistic bodywork and physical therapy (myotherapy, global postural reeducation, microkinesiology) and massage (energetic, metamorphic, lymphatic, foot reflexology, Boysen's biodynamic massage)

Through his practice and various trainings (biodecoding, sensitive dance), he continues to extend his understanding and study on the synergy between the body, emotions, thought, energy, and consciousness.

He has created a holistic health approach, called bioharmony, that is based on the awakening of the body's innate awareness and its natural potential for synchronization.

He offers individual treatments in this method as well as group sessions and workshops. He is especially active in providing ongoing training to those interested in the use of touch for help and treatment, stress management, preventive care, and increasing bodily awareness. This training is offered to individuals working in the fields of health and social services, as well as business.

He is currently working on a follow-up book that will focus on energy and bioharmonic massage.

Trainings and Workshops

Information can be found at his office in Angers, France, or on his website. Currently he offers a five-day course in the use of touch for providing health treatment and assistance and a course in bioharmonic self-massages that takes place over three weekends. Possibilities are always available for those interested in ongoing training.

Contact

For more information on workshops and trainings, or if you wish to contact the author:

E-mail: espacecorporel@free.fr
Website: www.labioharmonie.com

INDEX

Page numbers in *italics* refer to figures.